Cover: The illustration is an 18th century engraving of distillation apparatus for producing ether in a London laboratory.

Nepenthe refers to a mythical medicine which brings relief from 'pains and irritations', and induces forgetfulness, as described in the 8th century BC in Homer's *Odyssey* (Chapter Two).

NEPENTHE'S CHILDREN

THE HISTORY OF THE DISCOVERIES OF MEDICINES FOR SLEEP AND ANESTHESIA

Wallace B. Mendelson

Pythagoras Press

New York

About the Author

Wallace B. Mendelson, MD is Professor of Psychiatry and Clinical Pharmacology (ret) at the University of Chicago. He is a Distinguished Fellow of the American Psychiatric Association and a member of the American Academy of Neuropsychopharmacology. He has been director of the Section on Sleep Studies at the National Institute of Mental Health, the Sleep Disorders Center at the Cleveland Clinic Foundation, and the Sleep Research Laboratory at the University of Chicago. He is the author of nine books and numerous professional papers involving sleep and pharmacology. His many research interests over the years have included a number of drugs involved in anesthesia in the present or past, including propofol, benzodiazepines, and barbiturates. He has been recognized with the Academic Achievement Award from the American Sleep Disorders Association in 1999 and an award for excellence in sleep and psychiatry from the National Sleep Foundation in 2010. More information about Dr. Mendelson and his work is available in Wikipedia at https://en.wikipedia.org/wiki/Wallace_B._Mendelson and on his website at http://zhibit.org/wallacemendelson.

Disclaimer and Conflict of Interest Statement

CONFLICT OF INTEREST: Dr. Mendelson has no financial arrangements with any pharmaceutical company marketing any medicines mentioned in this book.

DISCLAIMER: This book contains information on a variety of illnesses as well as their treatments. It is not a substitute for medical evaluation and treatment. If you believe you have any of the illnesses mentioned in this book, please consult your doctor.

TABLE OF CONTENTS

PROLOGUE

Life had not been easy for William Morton. In 1836 when he was seventeen, money had disappeared from the till at the tavern where he worked, and the sheriff of Worcester, Massachusetts had run him out of town. Then there had been the matter of bad checks and false entries in the ledgers of his dry goods business in Rochester. Even his church had expelled him for dishonesty. He had barely made it out of Cincinnati, leaving a trail of bad debts, and where his illicitly acquired U.S. Mail seals had been used to backdate business documents. Then there had been the accusations of embezzling in Washington, DC.

But things were starting to settle down now. He had gone to dental school, returned to his hometown in Massachusetts, and then met a dentist named Horace Wells, who continued to teach him the trade. He became engaged to a lovely young lady, a congressman's niece named Elizabeth Whitman. In order to appease her family, who preferred someone with a more prestigious profession, he enrolled in medical school. He dropped out after the marriage, but not before having heard Dr. Charles Jackson speak of the possibilities of inhaling the evaporating gas from a sweet-smelling liquid for anesthesia. Now he was on his own. Dr. Wells had tossed him out of their practice where he made dentures, saying he lacked the needed skill, as well as a small matter of missing funds. On September 30, 1846 he administered the gas when doing a tooth extraction and it seemed to ease the patient's pain. Maybe this was his big break. On October 1, he talked with an attorney about patenting the gas, disguising its origin and smell with tincture of orange. Then, on October 16, 1846, he planned to demonstrate to the doctors at Massachusetts General Hospital, whose main medicines for anesthesia were opium or alcohol, that his gas—ether—could alleviate the pain of surgery. The demonstration was successful[1]. Word rapidly spread in the medical community, and this revolutionary development changed the practice of surgery from an excruciating race against the clock to a more tolerable and less painful process[2].

The story of anesthetic gases goes back much further, and continued much later, than the clinical discovery of ether. One thread extends back to the 7th century BC in ancient Greece:

In the temple of Apollo on the slopes of Mount Parnassus, an older woman, the Pythia, sat on a tripod seat in a sacred chamber. Beneath her, from a crack in the rock, rose gases, thought to emanate from the body of a huge python slain by Apollo in the mythical past. Intoxicated by the gases, and perhaps other substances such as oleander, the Pythia made rambling, ecstatic pronouncements, which were interpreted by the priests into prophecies for the kings who had traveled from all over the known world to seek her advice about their difficulties.

Two and a half millennia later, in 1908, the botanists at the University of Chicago botanical gardens had their own problems. Ever since they had installed illuminating gas fixtures in the greenhouses, the carnation flowers were wilting. It turned out that the culprit was ethylene, part of the gas derived from coal tar, which itself came from ancient organisms. Some years later, physiologists Arno Luckhardt and J. Bailey Carter tried to clarify its properties. When they exposed animals to ethylene, they became unconscious. Inhaling it themselves, Luckhardt and Carter had the same experience. Realizing its potential, they made a prophecy of their own: ethylene might become a useful anesthetic for humans. It turned out that their prediction was correct. After testing it for safety and then gaining experience with 106 operations, they published the results in 1923 and later turned it over to the profession without patenting it. Ethylene became a widely used surgical anesthetic for several decades.

In this book, we will look at how ether, ethylene, and many other anesthetic or sleep-inducing substances which came before and after them were discovered. Before we turn to these medicines, though, in the following Introduction we will talk about anesthesia and sleep, both their similarities as well as their differences.

INTRODUCTION: SLEEP AND ANESTHESIA—DISTANT COUSINS

Anesthesia refers to a loss of sensation. General anesthesia is a drug-induced reversible state which provides relief from pain along with a number of other qualities desirable for surgery: unconsciousness, immobility in response to stimuli, and later amnesia for the experience. Other desirable qualities are muscle relaxation, and inhibition of a reflex response to surgery in which blood pressure and heart rate can become excessive.

As we will see in Chapter One, early attempts to reach some of these goals involved plant-based substances, which induce intoxication, a poor substitute for anesthesia. Alcohol and opiates, used since ancient times, can potentially provide anesthesia, but only in quantities that are on the edge of toxicity which can easily become lethal. The heroic cowboy depicted in movies taking a drink of whiskey before a bullet is extracted was likely to be intoxicated, but to still experience significant pain.

Even in modern times, no single medicine fully provides reliable prolonged clinical anesthesia. Intravenous barbiturates, for instance, induce unconsciousness, but do not prevent movement in response to surgical activity, indicating that stimuli are still perceived. Neuromuscular blocking drugs can cause immobility, but do not provide unconsciousness or prevent pain. Most newer inhaled agents produce unconsciousness and immobility, but in anesthetic doses have little effect by themselves on reducing pain. Modern anesthesia, then, is accomplished usually by a combination of several types of agents: an intravenous sedative-hypnotic agent to begin the process ('induction'), a muscle relaxant, the newer inhaled anesthetics such as sevoflurane to maintain anesthesia, and medication for pain.

In contrast to general anesthesia, sleep is a naturally occurring, universal process involving reversible quiescence, unconsciousness, and reduced responsiveness to one's surroundings. [3] Unlike anesthesia, a sleeping person usually can be awakened by outside stimuli such as sound and touch. Sleep is also influenced by body clock mechanisms ('circadian rhythms') and a homeostatic process which strives to keep one's total amount of sleep relatively constant over time[4].

Studies of brainwaves ('the electroencephalogram, or EEG') and other measures reveal that it is made up of two major states, rapid eye movement (REM) sleep as well as NREM sleep, which in turn is made up of three stages. REM and NREM sleep are very actively regulated by the nervous system, alternating across the course of the night in an approximately ninety-minute cycle in humans, and the amount of the particular stages in NREM sleep vary across the night depending on how long one has been asleep and the circadian time

Sleep and anesthesia are similar in the sense that they both involve unconsciousness, and are reversible; that is, a person spontaneously awakens from sleep, and recovers from anesthesia when the medicines are stopped. This is in contrast to coma, in which unconsciousness and unresponsiveness, often stemming from brain injury, are very marked and potentially very long lasting[5]. But sleep and anesthesia also differ in a number of ways. A person can be aroused from sleep by sensory stimulation, but not during ongoing anesthesia. In most forms of general anesthesia, the brainwaves in deeper levels tend to be large, slow 'delta' waves[6]; however, the EEG does not have the dynamic, cyclic processes of sleep stages, and no equivalent to the REM-NREM sleep cycle.[i] Sleep is also unlike general anesthesia in that during normal sleep, although there are fluctuations in blood pressure and respiration (especially in REM

---

[i] Since the 1930s, there has been a concept of stages or phases of anesthesia, which include induction, a transient period of excitement, surgical anesthesia, and overdose. These are not stages in the sense in which we are using the word in relation to sleep— actively regulated, cyclic patterns of the EEG and other physiologic processes. The concept of stages of anesthesia was developed during the age of ether being given alone for anesthesia, and to a significant degree involves observation of muscle activity, including muscles of respiration. In the modern age in which muscle relaxants and intravenous induction agents are used as part of a combination of drugs for anesthesia, the utility of the concept is thought by many to be less clear; there is more emphasis now on physiologic measures of responsiveness, circulation, and respiration as indicators of depth of anesthesia.

sleep) in healthy individuals, these processes are basically preserved[ii]; in general anesthesia this is not the case.

Some anesthetics produce many of their effects through brain regions involved in sleep regulation, though they may not necessarily do so in a similar manner as in naturally occurring sleep[7]. Because of the superficial resemblance of being a state of unconsciousness and unresponsiveness, it is common for anesthesiologists to explain to patients that they will be going to sleep or some similar phrase, but because of the differences in the two processes, this is not really accurate, but should be understood as a metaphor.[iii]

Though sleep and anesthesia differ in many ways, one thing they have in common is that from the dawn of history people have tried to use drugs to manipulate them. As we have described, sleep is actively regulated in a complex manner. When this highly orchestrated process goes awry, the result is the experience of insomnia, resulting in difficulty going to sleep or staying asleep. Over the millennia, dozens of kinds of substances have been used in an attempt to return sleep to its normal restful state, just as there have been a wide range of substances given in an effort to produce

---

[ii] The exception to this is, of course, some sleep disorders, notably central and obstructive sleep apnea.

[iii] In much the same way, sleep is often used as a euphemism for death, as in Shakespeare's *Hamlet*, in which Horatio says to the dead Hamlet: 'Good night, sweet prince. May hosts of angels sing you to sleep...'

anesthesia. The histories of the compounds used for these purposes are deeply intertwined. From the earliest days, for instance, alcohol has been used, not very successfully, for both purposes. Moving ahead to the 19th century, the inhaled anesthetic chloroform led to the creation of the first synthetic sleeping pill, chloral hydrate. In many cases, the drugs which are now used intravenously for the induction process, and which are also used in waking sedation for medical procedures, are the same compounds which have been developed as orally administered tranquilizers and sleeping pills ('hypnotics'). Often the difference is primarily dose and method of administration. Moving ahead to more recent times, for instance, the benzodiazepine midazolam came onto the market in Europe as an oral sleeping pill, and was widely thought to cause minimal memory disturbance in the morning; on the other hand, it is used intravenously for conscious sedation or anesthesia induction with the perceived advantage of providing amnesia for uncomfortable medical procedures. Because their stories are so interconnected, in this book we will describe how both types of drugs developed together, first as natural plant products and later as chemically synthesized medicines, from the earliest times until the mid-to-late 20th century.

Why focus on this time period? One reason is that at this point the medicines in the two fields became more specialized, but another is that around then there began to be a change in the way hypnotics and anesthetics were developed. Starting with halothane in 1951, the growing complexity and resources needed for large screening procedures and what came to be known as rational drug design (Chapter Six) were such that the story of discoveries gradually became more one of industries, and not as much of individuals. Halothane, for instance, as well as its predecessor trichloroethylene, were products of group efforts at Imperial Chemical Industries, a conglomeration of four chemical companies, and for a long time the biggest manufacturer in the U.K., producing nylon, polyester, plastics, non-ferrous metals, dyestuffs, and herbicides. This process comes from a long and important trend, the evolution of organic chemistry, beginning with the synthetic dye industry in the mid-19th century, and evolving into a wide range of products including medicines, food coloring, paints, fertilizers, explosives, and other products.[8] As such, the story of halothane and the later volatile anesthetics, though invaluable to the modern practice of anesthesia, marked the end of an era in which remarkable individuals, in many cases working outside of either academia or industry, stumbled upon new drugs which revolutionized medical care. One of the discoverers of chloroform, for instance, was a rural family doctor with a homemade laboratory, who came across it while distilling whiskey and chlorinated lime to make a pesticide, and became aware of its hypnotic qualities by accident (Chapter Two). Ether became clinically used because of the complicated interactions of a shady dentist with a history of forgery, a patrician Harvard professor who also believed he had taught Samuel Morse the secret of the telegraph, and a Connecticut dentist who was later arrested for throwing acid on prostitutes (also Chapter Two). One of the goals of this book is to describe the discovery of drugs in an era when creative individuals, warts and all, and often aided by chance, played a relatively large role, before the advent of organized teams backed by large resources and guided by rational drug design. As we benefit today from high-tech processes in which thousands of compounds are routinely screened for potential as medicines, I believe it is also important that we don't forget this earlier, haphazard, and colorful time.

The interested reader will also find a postscript, which for the sake of completeness briefly summarizes the subsequent development of drugs for sleep and anesthesia to the present day. This also relates to a second goal, which is to make this story accessible and provide a sense of perspective to the reader who does not have a technical background, but who is curious where medicines came from. For this reason, I have tried to make the body of the text interesting and understandable to the general reader, while providing footnotes for those who would like to pursue more specialized information. It is hoped that this book will also be interesting to students and trainees in the medical sciences who would like to learn more about how their fields came to be where they are today.

CHAPTER ONE: FROM PREHISTORIC TIMES THROUGH THE MEDICAL RENAISSANCE

Prehistory: Alkaloids— 'chemical thorns' and the earliest psychoactive agents

The origins of drugs which cause unconsciousness—and indeed all psychoactive drugs—lie in the history of how plants and species which prey upon them, whether bacteria, insects or animals, evolved together. Typically, this happened by one developing protective measures, then the other coming to have countermeasures, followed by a new protective adaptation in the first one, in an ongoing cycle. The process by which two interacting species produce genetic change in each other, known as coevolution, is thought to be a major driver in biological diversity. Among the ways in which plants can form defenses are growing thorns, for instance. If animals find ways of dealing with them, another plant response can be producing alkaloids, nitrogen-containing substances which may have various physiologic functions including acting as 'chemical thorns,' with unpleasant smell or taste, or which produce toxicity. In some cases, these could take the form of naturally occurring pesticides. Alternatively, in responding to mammals, plants may produce chemicals which result in experiences which are unpleasant, lower ability for vigilance or defense due to intoxication or sedation, or which are biologically toxic. Examples include strychnine, psilocin, cocaine, morphine, nicotine, and perhaps several thousand others.

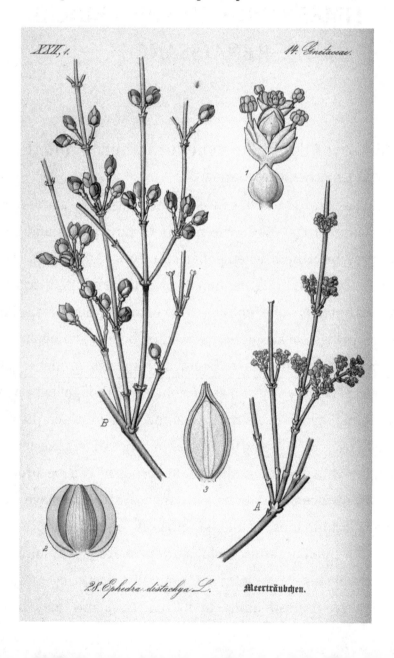

Figure 1-1: Ephedra distachya. *Extracts of plants from the genus* Ephedra *containing ephedrine were used in Chinese medicine as early as the Han Dynasty (206 BC-220 AD) for asthma. In the West, jumping ahead two millennia, ephedrine was the active ingredient in Vick's nose drops for congestion, which came on the market in 1948. The synthetic form is still used today to reduce excessive secretions during surgery (Chapter Four).*

Our ancestors, then, were faced with a large assortment of substances produced by plants or fungi, which could affect them in a variety of ways. Some writers have speculated that stories which appear in many cultures associating eating apples or other fruits with paradise may reflect ancient experiences with psychoactive substances[9]. Plants containing substances that alter consciousness, many of which evolved over millennia into medicines, were abundant in pre-history. The poppy originated in Lower Mesopotamia (Southwest Asia), and Sumerians referred to it as early as 3400 BC as Hul Gil, the 'joy plant.' Solanaceous plants[iv] containing potent alkaloids such as henbane, mandrake, and datura were found in the Middle and Far East as well as Europe. In what would later be called the New World, the coca bush had been found in the Andes since the 3rd century BC.

[iv] Solanaceous flowering plants refer to the nightshade family, known for their alkaloids, but also including food crops such as potatoes, tomatoes, peppers, and eggplant.

The unhappy goat of Azazel: Drugs in magic and religion

Many of these substances found their way into the practice of primitive religions. Much of the history of developing medicines for sleep and anesthesia involves the later extrication of this association. Lest this be considered an issue only of prehistoric times, one need only remember the 19th century attacks against James Young Simpson's use of chloroform as an obstetric anesthetic, on the grounds that it opposed the biblical dictum that childbirth involved suffering (Chapter Two), or the 'Salvarsan Wars' in the early 20th century, accusing Paul Ehrlich, the developer of a major drug for syphilis, of encouraging sin

In hunter-gatherer societies, affirmation of being part of a group was reinforced by ingesting plant products supplied by a shaman, in which inebriation resulted in experiences which seemed to give knowledge of the world and one's place in it[10]. Diseases were looked upon as punishments or signs of impurity, and one major way of healing was to transfer them to a sacrificial person or animal. The word 'scapegoat' itself is derived from a Hebrew word meaning 'goat for Azazel.' Leviticus 16:8-10 describes how once a year a goat was selected, and the hapless animal was hurled off a cliff in an effort to cleanse the people of their sins in the eyes of the fallen angel Azazel. Another later approach was to engage in symbolic sacrifices in the agape (sacramental banquet) in which one would ingest representations of a sacrificial god, often in the form of an alcoholic drink or peyote or fungus products[11]. With the beginnings of availability of nutritious grains and edible grapes, and hence the beginning of farming settlements, in the Neolithic period (roughly 9000-3000 BC depending on the area), the tradition of sacrifice continued to evolve over the centuries.

Some historians have suggested that the use of medicines became entwined over time with the practice of sacrifice. The Greek word *phármakon,* from which we derive 'pharmacy' and 'pharmacology' is similar to *pharmakós,* referring to the practice of transferring guilt to a scapegoat figure[12]. One festival of Apollo in ancient Greece, known as Thargelia, honored the first fruits and wheat crop of May or June. In the process, a particularly ugly or deformed person was selected as the *pharmakoi.* He or she was first fed well, then beaten with vegetation (hence shifting any uncleanliness in the crop to them), including ritualistically whipping the genitals with fig branches seven times. They were run out of town, or in more desperate times, the unlucky scapegoat might be stoned, hurled into the sea, or burned. Later, as Greek society evolved, this practice is thought to have been the basis for the 5th century BC practice of ostracism, in which once a year citizens would vote to select an individual, who was not necessarily accused of wrongdoing, to leave within ten days, and not return for ten years.

Even beyond the association of sacrifice, we still see the origins involving magic in our words for medicines and pharmacists. The Greek word *phármakon* refers not only to a drug, but also charms, philters, or enchantment, and a *pharmakeus* was "a preparer of drugs, a poisoner, a sorcerer."[13]

The classical period in ancient Greece

In Greece during the Age of Pericles (495-429 BC), healing, magic, and medicines remained intertwined. In the temples of Asclepius, supplicants were bathed and purified, then ingested substances, presumably hallucinogens, which led them to experience 'temple sleep.' In this state they would have healing dreams, in which Asclepius or his daughters would come to them and advise them on what would be necessary for getting better. As we mentioned in the Prologue, the Pythia, or oracle, at the Temple of Apollo at Delphi would breathe vapors from underground, which might have been ethylene (later to be used as a surgical anesthetic in the 1920s; see Chapter Three) or methane. In legend, the gas itself was supposed to result from the remains of a great serpent, slain by the god Apollo and thrown into a crevice from which the fumes emanated. Alternatively, the oracle might also have chewed on oleander leaves containing conessine, a steroid histamine antagonist, as well as oleandrin, a toxic cardiac glycoside. In the resultant trance-like state, the oracle would make prophecies, which rulers from all of Greece would come to hear. In the Dionysian Mysteries, secret cult ceremonies in honor of the god of wine, theater, and religious ecstasy, followers would ingest a drink known as Kykeon. It was made from water, *Glechon* (a plant genus in the mint family), and barley, the latter containing an ergot fungus producing a hallucinatory substance. The resulting intoxication, accompanied by music and dancing, was thought to result in an uninhibited state of religious exultation.

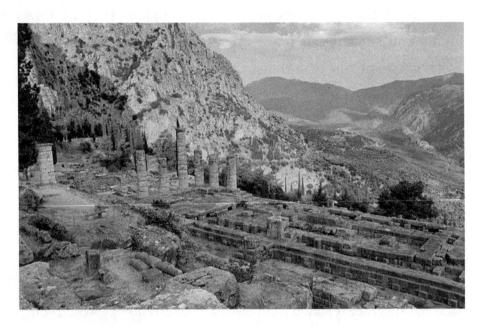

Figure 1-2: *Part of the temple of Apollo at Delphi, from the 4ᵗʰ century BC. Shrines at this site go back much earlier, starting from a small structure of woven laurel, then one which legend says was constructed of beeswax and feathers, then of bronze, and finally of stone. In ancient times, an oracle, intoxicated by naturally formed gases and possibly alkaloids, made pronouncements which were interpreted as predictions or aids to important decisions, which were highly valued.*

The culture of the time also associated drugs with magic and witchcraft. In *The Odyssey*, Homer's epic poem dating back to the late bronze age in 8ᵗʰ century BC but a cultural foundation of classical Greek life, the goddess/sorceress Circe transforms Odysseus' men into swine by giving them extracts of the solanaceous plants mandrake and possibly datura, both of which contain potent alkaloids. She also is said to have poisoned the water in which a romantic rival bathed, changing her into a very un-lovely shape, not to mention having converting Picus, an Italian king who was immune to her charms, into a woodpecker. She was known as a *polypharmakos*, one who knows many drugs, and all in all, a person not to be trifled with.

This was the cultural context into which stepped Hippocrates of Kos (c460-c370 BC), sometimes known as the 'father of medicine.' While working as an Asclepiad, a physician and teacher from a medical family who was neither a temple priest nor part of a physicians' guild[14], he came up with a revolutionary idea about the nature of diseases. Instead of being a punishment from on high, dealt with by sacrifice, diseases resulted from disorders of physiology which could be treated directly. Though Hippocrates' work was limited by long-outgrown notions such as the role of the humors (blood, phlegm, yellow and black bile) it was a first step in changing the understanding of how to approach human illness.

Hippocrates' new view of diseases led as well to a new way of looking at medicines, which he believed were not supernatural. They were derived from plants, and in his view had understandable interactions with the body. Unlike foods, which were overcome by the body and transformed for its needs, drugs instead overcame the body and induced changes in it. The importance of dose was recognized, and indeed the general belief was that the only difference between a drug and a poison was the amount administered. In view of the widespread use of opiates both recreationally and in medicines, it is not surprising that the notion of tolerance also developed. It was reasoned that these drugs gained their potency from lack of familiarity to the body; with growing familiarity, they became less powerful.

Hippocrates believed that opium did not have magical properties, but described it as useful as a hypnotic, for pain, and for what he believed were uterine disorders. He recommended extracts of juniper (*Juniperus macrocarpa*) for pain and chills related to childbirth. Spearmint (*Mentha spicata*) was used as a diuretic, to reduce nausea, and to decrease anxiety. Pomegranate (*Punica granatum*) fruit rind served as an antidiarrheal and for treatment for parasites. Mandrake (*Mandragora*), sometimes known as 'Circe's root,' was widely used in Greek and Roman medicine, and the dream-like state and partial amnesia it seemed to produce was recommended for those undergoing surgery. Hippocrates also used the words analgesia and anesthesia, the latter apparently referring to disease-caused loss of sensation, and he noted that unconscious persons are less sensitive to pain.[15]

Witches and sorcerers: Beyond the classical period

Although some physicians persevered in using medicines from this viewpoint, the Romans and their successors often continued to intertwine medicines with religion and magic. This persisted into the

Middle Ages, when the practice of witchcraft included the use of draughts or ointments, which were thought to lead to otherworldly, and often erotic, experiences, as well as philters, or love potions. Self-styled witches and sorcerers were the dispensers of medicines including opiates and belladonna-related substances from solanaceous plants for healing purposes. Not surprisingly, their administration of medicines was among their crimes as seen in the eyes of the Inquisition

There were also those who persisted in studying medicines in a non-magical, non-religious context. They gained support from the returning Crusaders, who described the skills of Arab physicians, who often prescribed psychoactive substances. The re-discovery by alchemists of distillation, long known in the Arab world, made possible the use of tinctures with high alcohol content.

For those who wished to study and dispense medicines, it became vital to avoid the hazards of the Inquisition by distinguishing their activities from those of magicians. One way to do this was by practicing their professions inside the newly formed institution of universities, which began to appear, for instance, in Bologna (1088), Paris (1150), and Oxford (1167). The packaging of the medicines themselves was redesigned so that they did not resemble those used in magic—ointments, for instance, were often replaced by pills and tinctures. The *spongia somnifera*, with roots going back much further, began to be used in surgery. It consisted of a cloth impregnated with opium, mandrake, henbane, and hemlock, through which a patient breathed. Afterwards, vapor from vinegar was used to initiate arousal.

In summary, through the 1400s, patients undergoing surgery were generally given intoxicants or sedatives, usually opium as well as alcohol, often in combination with henbane, mandragora, or other substances. This remained the case until the clinical appearance of the first general anesthetics such as ether in the 19th century. Beginning in the 1500s, though, new ways of approaching medicines began to appear, in the form of the Medical Renaissance.

'The universities do not teach all things.': Paracelsus and the Medical Renaissance

A leader in the new movement was Paracelsus (1493-1541), born Theophrastus von Hohenheim, who rejected the writings of the ancients and the teachings at the universities in favor of the experience of his contemporary apothecaries, barber-surgeons, and sorcerers. The son of a physician, as a youth he followed the common practice of traveling around Europe from teacher to teacher. Never one to be modest about his accomplishments, after getting degrees from the University of Vienna in 1510 and Ferrara in 1516, he renamed himself Paracelsus (as great or greater than Aulus Cornelius Celsus, a famous classical Roman physician and writer).

After graduation, he continued his wanderings, including time as a military surgeon, where his exploits included capture and escape from the Tartars in Russia. He taught at the University of Basel from 1526 to 1528, where he scandalized his colleagues by wearing an alchemist's apron instead of academic regalia, and lecturing in German instead of Latin. He is perhaps best known for his disdain for authorities, and in 1527 nailed up an announcement of his lectures and an invitation to all (not just academics) to attend; a few weeks later on St. John's Day, he publicly burned the books of the well-known Arab physician Avicenna as well as the classical Greek Galen. These actions have reminded some of Martin Luther, who had nailed his Theses to the church door in Wittenberg Castle ten years previously, and later burned a papal bull. Though Paracelsus himself denied a similarity, his emphasis on turning from authorities to the wisdom of experience of the common man brings the comparison to mind.

Not long after the book burning, and perhaps not coincidentally the death of a prestigious patient, Paracelsus took up again his life as an itinerant physician. After publishing *Der grossen Wundartzney ('The Great Surgery Book'),* his prestige grew once again, and he became a wealthy man. He died in 1541, under somewhat mysterious conditions, at an inn in Salzburg.

Paracelsus believed that 'the universities do not teach all things' and there was much to be learned from people with extensive experience but no formal academic background. Among these, he believed were 'gipsies, sorcerers, wandering tribes, old robbers and such outlaws.'[16] As had Hippocrates, he emphasized the importance of dose, which often distinguished drugs from poisons. He was among the first to look for medicines for specific illnesses, instead of grand panaceas thought to help all disorders. Although he subscribed to his own theory of humors, he also recognized that illnesses could be brought about by the body being afflicted by outside agents.

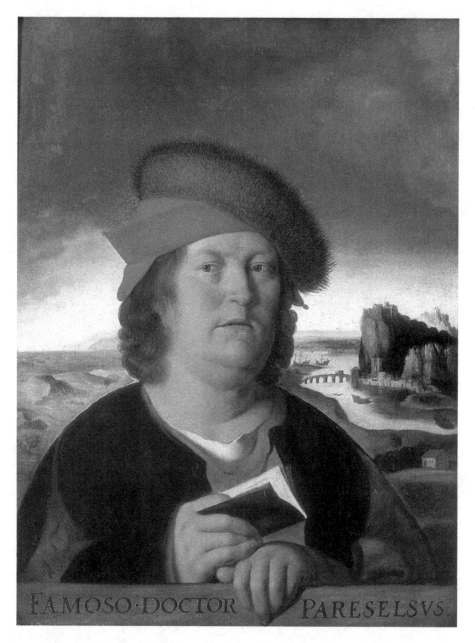

Figure 1-3: *A depiction of Paracelsus, one of many 17th century copies of the lost original by the Flemish painter Quentin Matsys (1456/1466-1530).*

At one point, Paracelsus experimented with ether in animals, though he did not bring this to a human level. His preference was for the laudanum which he developed, a tincture of opium which he believed had many uses. He recommended ingestion of mercury for syphilis, and antimony for its purgative effects. The first pharmacopoeias, clearly influenced by his work, began to appear in Nuremberg (1546) and Basle (1561), and contained belladonna-related compounds often in combination with opiates, many of them derived from witches' formulations. The English physician Thomas Sydenham (1624-1689) continued this tradition with a mixture which included opiates, wine cloves, cinnamon, and saffron. A hint of magical associations remained, in the practice of combining opiates with powders made from pearls, jade, or gold.

All of this was part of what came to be known as the Medical Renaissance, which occurred from the early 1500s until about 1700. It involved respect for the ancient Greeks and Romans, but also new discoveries and the medical knowledge of the Arabs and Persians. The latter was made available in Spain and Sicily, which continued to have large Arab populations, though re-conquered by Christians since the 11th century. Like the Renaissance in general, it involved a move toward humanism and away from medieval scholasticism, which had emphasized reasoning and drawing inferences from the classics, as well as rationalizing Christianity with the ancient Greek writings. Ultimately, the Medical Renaissance marked a decline in the Church's authority over medical training and university life. Major figures included Leonardo da Vinci (1452-1519), whose art was influenced by his studies of the eye, and how visual information was transferred by the optic nerve to the brain. Others included Ambrose Paré (1510-1590), a French physician who made advances in surgical methods and wound care, the Flemish anatomist Andreas Vesalius (1514-1564), who produced elaborate drawings of humans based on dissections, and the English physician William Harvey (1578-1657), who emphasized and quantified the process of blood circulation. This new spirit provided the backdrop for the later discovery of new medicines.

CHAPTER TWO: FROM PLANT-BASED INTOXICANTS TO ETHER, CHLOROFORM, AND THE FIRST SYNTHETIC HYPNOTICS (THE 18th AND 19th CENTURIES)

An intoxicating experience: Cannabis, alkaloids, alcohol, opiates

As a result of the change in approach represented by the Medical Renaissance and the developments of the next centuries, by the late 18th and early 19th centuries the choices for surgical anesthesia were numerous but limited in effectiveness.

Cannabis as an anesthetic: Cannabis was used for anesthesia as far back as 600 BC by the great Indian surgeon Sushruta, and later mixed with wine in surgical procedures by Hua Tuo (140-208 AD), a Chinese physician in the time of the Han Dynasty. Widely used recreationally in the West, and given for other purposes such as wound dressing, ear pain, nausea, and fever reduction, overall, historically it had less medical impact than in the East. Though brought to the attention of Western medicine in the 1830s by William Brooke O'Shaughnessy for intestinal disorders, muscle spasms, and pain, and by others for headaches, sleep, and seizure disorders, this apparently did not extend in any substantial way to use in surgical anesthesia, and has not in subsequent years. On a related topic, in recent years there has been growing awareness that recreational cannabis use before surgery can alter the anesthesia process, including requiring higher doses of propofol for induction[17].

Currently, although medical marijuana is not approved by the U.S. Food and Drug Administration for any specific medical purpose, some prescription cannabinoids have been approved for two rare forms of infantile and childhood epilepsy, loss of appetite in HIV, and nausea during chemotherapy. There is active research for possible uses in psychiatric illness, as well as skin and eye diseases and autoimmune disorders. A recent review of research suggests that some plant-based and prescription cannabinoids may have benefits in chronic pain; studies of acute pain have had mixed outcomes, and reports in postoperative pain have been negative[18].

Difficulty sleeping is one of the common motivations (along with anxiety and pain) for seeking medical marijuana. The data on sleep effects are mixed, depending on dose, and whether one is looking at whole-plant cannabis, its constituent 'cannabinoids' (including THC, which produces the euphoriant effects of marijuana, and CBD, which is not psychoactive), or synthetic related compounds. Different types of marijuana and localities where it is grown also vary widely in their composition and relative amounts of cannabinoids, adding to the variability of results. In general, studies of THC on sleep have varied from negative findings[19] to reports of decreased time to fall asleep[20] in both normal sleepers and persons with sleep difficulty, often with increases in stage N3 (slow-wave sleep) and decreases in REM. In contrast to the sedative effects of THC, CBD may be alerting, with increased awakenings during the night. Cannabinoids are not approved in the U.S. for helping sleep. A report by the U.S. National Academies/Institute of Medicine found moderate evidence of benefits from some cannabinoids (particularly nabiximols) for short-term outcomes in sleep-disturbance in some medical conditions such as fibromyalgia, multiple sclerosis, and chronic pain, but did not find available good-quality studies in chronic primary insomnia[21]. Interestingly, some synthetic cannabinoids have been reported to benefit obstructive sleep apnea in the short term[22].

Studies of whole-plant cannabis have varied; in chronic pain patients there are some data that it may decrease awakenings during the night in the short term, but that longer-term use might result in more difficulties going to sleep, as well as increased awakenings.[23] The observation of falling asleep sooner when taken once but producing sleep disturbance in chronic use is a theme we will see again with alcohol.

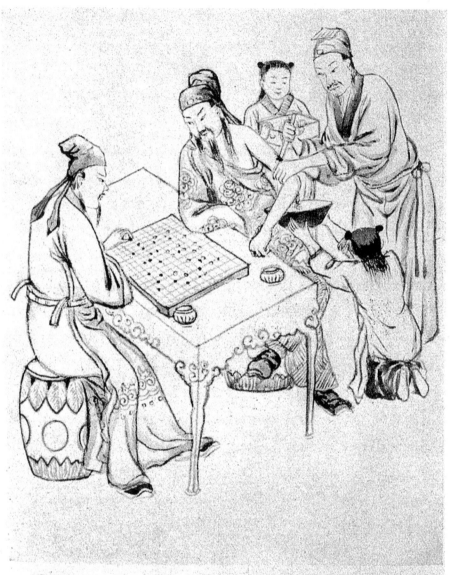

Surgeon HUA T'O operating upon the war hero KUAN KUNG for necrosis of arm resulting from a wound in battle. To detract his attention, chess (*wei-ch'i* 圍棋) is being played.

(Chinese painting)

Figure 2-1: *The Chinese physician Hua Tuo (140-208 AD) operating on the arm of the wounded war hero Kuan Kung. The patient is playing chess in order to turn his attention from the surgery. Hua Tuo was also an advocate of giving patients cannabis in wine.*

Plant alkaloids: Henbane had been used by the Babylonians as far back as 2250 BC for toothache. Pedanius Dioscorides (40-90 AD), a Greek physician who served in the Roman army, recommended mandrake in wine to produce insensibility for persons undergoing surgery. A major limitation, of course, was that its alkaloids could produce vomiting and diarrhea, hallucinations, and anticholinergic toxicity leading to death. Moreover, amounts of the active substances varied widely between different plants, seasons, and regions. Opiates, which we will talk about below, had been widely used in Europe for surgery since the 16th century, but were limited again by variation in potency across plants, and also by lack of an effective means of administration compatible with surgery. Ironically, in 1656, the architect Christopher Wren and chemist Robert Boyle had infused an opium/alcohol mixture intravenously into a dog using a goose quill and produced temporary anesthesia, but this was not pursued, and it was not until 1853 with the advent of an improved syringe that this began to be done in humans.

Alcohol: Alcohol [v] had of course been available since prehistoric times; its fumes had been tried for anesthesia since the

---

[v] The alcohols are a large family of compounds and are defined chemically as having a hydroxyl group (-OH) connected to a carbon atom in which all bonds are occupied. In this book we are using the word alcohol in its common usage as ethyl alcohol found in alcoholic beverages. There are many others, including the extremely toxic compounds methanol (which can cause permanent blindness) and isopropyl alcohol.

16th century, and direct ingestion since the 18th, but was generally unsatisfactory, because the amount needed approached or excessed toxicity and the duration of effect was often too brief. There were occasional reports of remarkable loss of pain sensation with oral alcohol; a Dr. Boott, one of the early advocates of ether, described the case of an Irishman whose alcoholic stupor was so great that while lying on the ground, he was unaware of a pig eating away portions of his face, which he only realized upon awakening. A surgeon at the Edinburgh Royal Infirmary described a drunken man who received a severe injury to the testicles, and underwent their later removal, without realizing it until after he was sober.[24] These were extreme cases, however, and most likely these unhappy drinkers were so inebriated that they were in the range of toxicity or coma, and not far from lethality. Typically, a person who drinks becomes intoxicated, a state very different from anesthesia, and in which pain can indeed be experienced. But the notion of intoxicating a patient, whether with alcohol or plant products such as mandrake or henbane, was clearly an impulse going back to ancient times, though largely dismissed once more modern anesthetics became available.

Oral alcohol is an unreliable sleep aid. When taken in the short term by persons who are not chronic users, it leads to falling asleep sooner; by the second half of the night, however, when blood concentrations have dropped, sleep becomes substantially disrupted, likely due to a kind of withdrawal response. At higher doses, REM sleep is decreased in the first half of the night, and in some studies increased in the second half. Total stage N3 (slow-wave sleep) tends to be increased at higher doses. The end result clinically is that any small benefits in going to sleep tend to be outweighed by the experience of disturbed sleep later at night.

In contrast to short-term use, alcohol dependent persons during chronic abstinence have very poor sleep, with decreased sleep efficiency, longer durations to fall asleep, and reduced slow-wave sleep.[25] These changes may last as long as two years after cessation of drinking. Poor sleep is sometimes the motivation for 'falling off the wagon' and returning to drink. In the very short term, alcohol may help in the sense that the time to fall asleep becomes shorter and slow-wave sleep may increase, but in the long term this perpetuates the significantly disrupted sleep of the alcohol-dependent person. Alcohol is also a respiratory depressant and can increase sleep-disturbed breathing in persons with sleep apnea.

Intravenous alcohol was used as far back as the 17th century, and the French physiologist Francois Magendie (1783-1855) reported using a combination of intravenous alcohol and camphor for cholera.[26] In the 1920s, there was some interest in giving intravenous alcohol for sedation and pain post-surgically, but this was largely abandoned due to complications such as damage to red blood cells and other side effects. There was some limited interest in various surgical and obstetrical purposes in the 1950s, but it is essentially no longer used. An intravenous preparation is still available for treating venous malformations, and it is sometimes used off-label for treating methanol or ethylene glycol poisoning. For the latter purpose, its mechanism is to compete with these agents for the enzyme which otherwise would break them down into toxic substances.

Opiates: Throughout this book we have described the use of opiates for pain, for instance, as advocated by Hippocrates in classical Greece, the *spongia somnifera* in Medieval times, and Paracelsus during the Medical Renaissance. It is the most likely candidate to be the ingredient in nepenthe, described in *The Odyssey* as the potent drug with which Helen of Troy sooths her troubled guests in Sparta:

> Then Helen, Zeus' daughter, thought of something else.
> She quickly dropped into the wine they were enjoying
> a drug which eased men's pains and irritations,
> making them forget their troubles. A drink of this,
> once mixed in with wine, would guarantee no man
> would let a tear fall on his cheek for one whole day,
> not even if his mother and his father died,
> or if, in his own presence, men armed with swords
> hacked down his brother or his son, as he looked on.[27]

Though these glittering words of praise seem very hopeful, in practice opiates have many drawbacks, not the least of which is dependence. In terms of sleep, the results are mixed. In patients with mild chronic pain, opioid use can increase the time to fall asleep.[28] When given acutely to 'post-addicts,' morphine has an arousing effect during sleep, increasing waking time, as well as decreasing slow-wave and REM sleep[29]. A similar study using computer-derived EEG measures reported that morphine and methadone increase arousal during sleep, with increased body movements and alpha EEG.[30] Opiates can also cause potentially fatal respiratory depression in persons with sleep apnea.

Sleep studies of chronic opiate use report a decrease in sleep efficiency and slow-wave sleep, as well as REM sleep.[31] Addicts typically describe difficulty going to sleep, awakenings during the night, and a sense that sleep was not restful, usually accompanied by daytime sleepiness. Thus, although opiates are potent behavioral sedatives and can produce a somnolent-like state, it may be appropriate that morphine is named after Morpheus, the god of dreams in Greek and Roman mythology, rather than Hypnos ('Somnus' in Latin), the god of sleep.

Opiates by themselves are also limited as anesthetics. As with alcohol, the doses required to provide all the needed qualities of anesthesia (including insensitivity to pain, unconsciousness and immobility, lack of reaction to stimuli, and muscle relaxation) approach or exceed toxic levels, which can lead to death from respiratory arrest or other causes. In modern general anesthesia, opiates continue to play an important role, but with lower doses in combination with other drugs for induction, maintenance, and muscle relaxation.

Going back to a historical perspective, though, by the early 1840s, the main anesthetics available to surgeons were alcohol and opiates. This is the setting in which the first inhalational anesthetics, nitrous oxide, ether, and chloroform, made their appearance.

Early inhalational anesthetics

Nitrous oxide— The laughing gas that financed Colt firearms: An early step along the road to inhaled anesthetics came with the work of Humphrey Davy (1778-1829), who rose from a modest background and training with a surgeon/apothecary to ultimately become the president of the Royal Society. Among his many interests—he was the discoverer of the elements calcium and magnesium—was the notion that healing gases could be used as treatments for consumption (tuberculosis). While experimenting on himself, Davy found that nitrous oxide, which had first been synthesized in 1772 by Joseph Priestley, had euphoric properties, as well as deadening the pain he was suffering from a toothache. In his 1800 book *Researches, Chemical and Philosophical,* he described its pain-relieving property and raised the idea that it might be employed in surgery, but these notions did not gain traction in the medical community. Laughing gas, as he called it, did find a place after 1799 as a recreational drug, particularly at parties of the well-to-do. Samuel Colt traveled for three years as the 'celebrated Dr. Coult of New York, London, and Calcutta,' administering laughing gas at fairgrounds for the audience's amusement in order to raise money for his fledgling firearms company[32]. George Poe, a cousin of

Edgar Allan Poe, was one of the first American commercial suppliers of nitrous oxide.

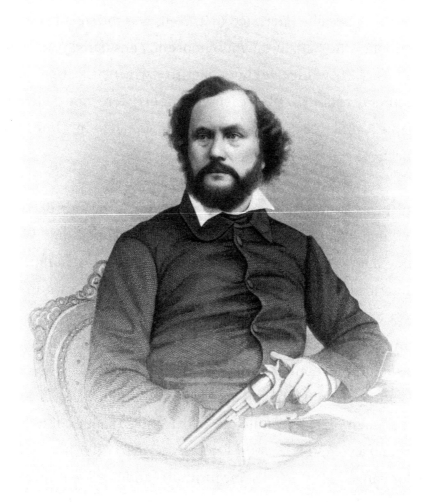

Figure 2-2: *Samuel Colt, in an 1855 steel engraving. At age 19, Colt built the first two models of his revolver, one of which wouldn't fire, while the other blew up. In order to raise money to try again, he traveled the fairgrounds, giving exhibitions of the intoxicating effects of nitrous oxide for entertainment. Ultimately he was able to hire a professional gunsmith to build a revolver based on his design, and founded his own company, now called Colt's Manufacturing Company.*

It wasn't until 1844 that the anesthetic properties of nitrous oxide were further explored, when an American dentist, Horace Wells (1815-1848), became interested in it. Wells was the son of farmers in Vermont, who initially taught school and considered going into the ministry. He ultimately chose dentistry, which he learned from an apprenticeship in 1834 (dental schools were not generally available until 1840) and began practicing in Hartford, Connecticut.

It had been known since Humphrey Davy's work four decades earlier that nitrous oxide had analgesic properties, but Wells became interested in its possible use in dentistry. At that time, as we described above, nitrous oxide was still mostly known in the context of recreation and entertainment of audiences. When the showman and medical school dropout Gardner Q. Colton put on an exhibition for entertainment in Hartford in December 1844, Wells attended with a dental application in mind. Colton's show was designed to demonstrate the intoxicating qualities of nitrous oxide, and a volunteer, Samuel Cooley, obliged. While intoxicated, Cooley banged his shin on some furniture, and Wells was quick to notice that he did not seem to feel the pain. Intrigued, he asked Colton for some nitrous oxide, and the next day inhaled it and felt no discomfort while his partner extracted a tooth. Enthused, he told his 25-year-old former apprentice and associate William T.G. Morton (1819-1868) about it, and Morton helped him arrange a demonstration in a public hall near Harvard Medical School in

January 1845. Something went wrong during a tooth extraction on a student, perhaps due to removing the gas bag too soon, and the patient cried out in pain. Critics labeled the use of nitrous oxide as 'humbug,' and Wells' reputation never recovered from the humiliation. By 1863, though, Gardner Q. Colton began using it successfully and with much publicity in dental clinics in New York and New Haven. It continues to be used by dentists to this day for mild sedation in combination with local anesthetics, and is used in obstetrics, but from early on it was recognized that it was not potent enough by itself for general surgery. There has also been interest in limiting its use because it contributes to depletion of ozone in the atmosphere.

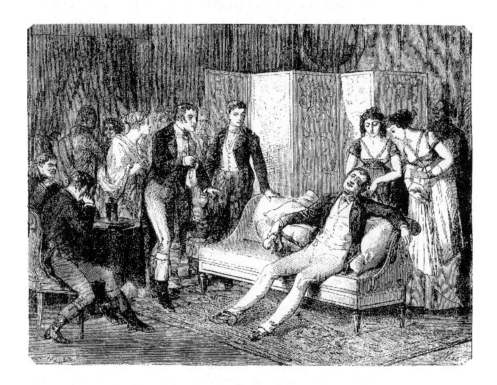

Figure 2-3: Humphry Davy's experiences breathing nitrous oxide at the Pneumatic Institute of Clifton, by Louis Figuler, 1868 (Author's translation). Davy experimented on himself and at various times gave nitrous oxide to eminent figures of the day such as the poets Samuel Taylor Coleridge and Robert Southey. James Watt, one of the inventors of the steam engine, became interested in respiratory techniques because of his son's tuberculosis, and he designed much of the equipment used by Davy.

Ether [vi] — A dubious dentist's dream of riches: The beginnings of ether lay in the Medical Renaissance when in 1540 the German physician Valerius Cordus (1515-1544) distilled alcohol and sulfuric acid ('oil of vitriol'), producing 'sweet oil of vitriol.' Paracelsus (Chapter One) reported its analgesic qualities in experiments with dogs, but it languished there until the 19th century. In 1818, Michael Faraday (1791-1867), the English scientist who among many other things advanced the understanding of electromagnetism and electrolysis, described its sedative and analgesic qualities. As with nitrous oxide, the medical profession showed little interest, but it became popular as an intoxicant at 'ether frolics' and was available in pubs. As it was known that people inhaling the sweet-smelling fumes described reduced pain, William T.G. Morton, a dentist with a shady past who had worked with Wells and knew his experience with nitrous oxide, experimented with ether on himself. He then gave ether to his patients and became

---

[vi] Ethers refer to a large group of compounds in which an oxygen atom is connected to two carbon atoms (technically, to what are known as alkyl or aryl groups). In this book, we are referring to diethyl ether, in common medical usage just referred to as 'ether.'

enthusiastic about its benefits. On October 16, 1846, on what later became known as 'Ether Day,' he gave a demonstration at Massachusetts General Hospital. The surgery, which was performed on a young man to remove a vascular neck tumor, was a success. Afterwards, the surgeon John Collins Warren famously, and possibly apocryphally, said, 'Gentlemen, this is no humbug.'

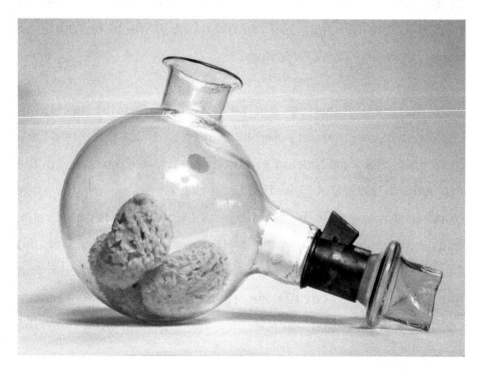

Figure 2-4: Morton's inhaler, including bottle for ether, valve which could be adjusted during surgery, and wooden mouthpiece.

The following day, Morton successfully administered ether during removal of a fatty tumor of the arm, and again on November 7 during a leg amputation. On November 21, Oliver Wendell Holmes, who had witnessed the first ether demonstration in Boston, wrote

Morton, suggesting the term 'anesthesia' (from the Greek word *anaisthesis*) and used as far back as Hippocrates[33] for the mental state induced by ether. He described it as a condition of insensibility, especially to the sense of touch. The Harvard surgeon Henry Jacob Bigelow (1818-1890) wrote a paper, 'Insensibility during surgical operations produced by inhalation,' which did much to bring ether to the attention of the medical world; in 2012, it was chosen by readers of the *New England Journal of Medicine* to be 'the most important article in *NEJM* history.'[34]

Here the medical success separated somewhat from the tale of exploiting its commercial possibilities. In retrospect, this might have been predicted from Morton's dubious past. As we described in the Prologue, at the age of 17 he had been caught stealing money while working at a tavern in his hometown of Charlton, Massachusetts, and he was told never to return. He moved on to Rochester and Cincinnati, where there were stories of falsified documents and other questionable activities. He apparently had a history of buying goods on credit, then after selling them disappearing with the money.

In 1840, he went to dental school in Baltimore, and after returning to Massachusetts in 1842, he met Wells, who became his mentor in an office in Hartford, Connecticut. In 1843, the two set up a joint practice in Boston, though Wells remained mostly in Hartford. Then in October 1844, Wells broke up the partnership, apparently both because he considered Morton not sufficiently skilled, as well as due to some funds which had disappeared. Undeterred, Morton opened his own office. In 1844, he also briefly attended Harvard Medical School, where he studied with Charles T. Jackson (1805-1880), a chemist and geologist, the son of a well-to-do ship owner and merchant in Plymouth, Massachusetts. Morton visited Jackson's laboratory, at which they apparently discussed ether. Morton dropped out of medical school, continuing his dental practice

In the first weeks after Ether Day, the 27-year-old Morton would not reveal what substance he had administered and took the unusual step of pursuing a patent for ether in combination with oil of orange. He called it 'Letheon,' referring to the River Lethe, the river of forgetfulness in Greek mythology. In the meantime, Jackson claimed that he had been the first to have had the idea of using ether in dentistry. He said that he had advised Morton to give it to dental patients in 1844. Morton's response was that he had been experimenting with ether anesthesia in animals before Jackson's suggestion, and that he had later visited Jackson's laboratory only to learn about the construction of his inhaler. In response to Jackson's claims of discovery, a deal was arranged so that he joined Morton on the patent, receiving 10 percent of profits, in comparison with Morton's 65 percent and the attorney's 25 percent. Since it was pretty clear that the active ingredient was the ether, the patent did them little good.

It also turned out that ether had been used in 1842 during surgery for a neck tumor by the Georgia physician Crawford W. Long (1815-

1878). Although Long continued to use ether, and indeed administered it to his wife during childbirth in 1845, he did not publish his work until 1849. He explained this delay by saying that he wished to have more patients to report, and he wanted to determine if there were other claims predating his own. He apparently had also had some concern that the lack of pain was due to the patient somehow mesmerizing himself, and he wished to gain enough experience to rule out this possibility. Long, who did make some efforts to receive credit, seems overall to have been less driven to gain fame for his work with ether, and he continued a distinguished career in surgery. He died, apparently of a stroke, in 1878, shortly after having administered ether to an obstetric patient. He appears to have been the only one involved in the ether controversy who went on to a successful and rewarding life. In 1920, the state of Georgia named a new county after him, as was the downtown teaching hospital of Emory University in 1931, until it was renamed in 2009.

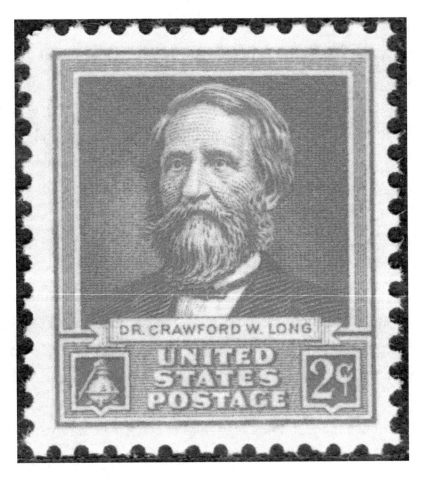

Figure 2-5: U.S. postage stamp honoring Dr. Crawford Long, 1940.

Things began to get more complicated. Jackson began gathering information about Morton's past improprieties. Morton petitioned Congress four times, requesting that it follow the European tradition of granting a reward to scientific discoveries. Both Jackson and Wells, claiming first discovery, lobbied against Morton's request for $100,000, which he never received.

Ultimately, none of the three were successful. Wells, who claimed to have given Morton the notion of inhalation of a gas for anesthesia, became very depressed after Morton's success and later experimented on himself with chloroform, to which he became addicted. He was later charged with splashing sulfuric acid onto a prostitute's shawl, and he committed suicide in jail. Jackson became more and more bitter. He had, it turned out, a history of disputing the work of others, going back to the 1820s, when he accused a Dr. Abraham Gesner of plagiarizing his paper on the geology of the Bay of Fundy. In 1840, he had contested Samuel Morse's patent of the telegraph, saying that he had given Morse the idea during a shipboard conversation in 1832, and he also believed that he had invented guncotton. In 1861, he published a book on ether, in which he said that he had taught Morton about ether anesthesia and led him to set up the demonstration on Ether Day. Unlike Morton, his family money made it possible for him to continue his career. Later, his behavior became erratic, and in 1873, he was admitted to McLean Asylum, where he died seven years later.

Morton's life, too, did not go as he (or others) expected. He gave little further clinical help with anesthesia to the surgeons at Massachusetts General Hospital (though he continued to rely on them for letters of support), and he didn't work on improvements in his system or encourage physicians to specialize in anesthesia. His focus seemed to be confined to the competitive advantage ether gave him in his dental practice, as well as capitalizing on ether through the patent or Congressional award, both of which ended badly. The notion of patenting, and profiting, from a process which would relieve pain for patients was offensive to many, and he came under vocal criticism. His efforts to gain recognition did not work out well. The state of Connecticut viewed Horace Wells as the discoverer of ether anesthesia. The French Academy of Sciences recognized Morton's contribution only in conjunction with Charles Jackson. He spent more and more of his time at his home (which he named Etherton) in Wellesley, Massachusetts in unrewarding efforts for publicity and dealing with his critics. In sum, the next twenty-one years after Ether Day were spent with progressive conflict, lack of the recognition he craved, and increasing financial difficulties due to the expenses of litigation about ether. In July 1868, he was upset by an article in the *Atlantic Monthly* which supported Jackson's claim to be the discoverer of ether anesthesia, and in order to challenge it he traveled to New York, which was experiencing a heat wave. While with his wife in a carriage in Central Park, he told the driver to stop. Apparently having a stroke, he became confused, saying that he was hot, and jumped into the lake. He was taken to St. Luke's Hospital, where he died at age 48.

Ether became widely used, particularly by the military. The first battlefield experiences with it were in the Mexican-American war of 1846-1848, and by 1849 army surgeons were formally supplied with it. Ultimately, it was largely replaced with the inhaled anesthetic chloroform, which was employed successfully in the Crimean War a few years later. In the American Civil War, both were used, but chloroform was preferred because it was easier to administer, more rapid in onset and not as flammable

Chloroform:

How a brew for pesticide became a surgical anesthetic: Chloroform, or trichloromethane, which is found in nature in small quantities as a product of seaweed and soil fungi, was synthesized at about the same time in 1831 by German chemist Justus von Liebig, the French pharmacist Eugene Soubeiran, and Samuel Guthrie, a doctor in rural northern New York State. Guthrie (1782-1848) had little formal training. He had briefly studied at New York's College of Physicians and Surgeons during the winter of 1810-1811 and spent a month at the University of Pennsylvania in 1813. Without a formal degree, he set up practice in Sackett's Harbor, a port city on Lake Ontario in northern New York, and as things were slow, engaged in a number of other activities. His work repairing firearms led to the invention of gunpowder 'percussion pills,' though in the process he was burned very badly in an explosion. Ultimately, though, the percussion pills contributed to the phasing out of flintlocks in favor of firearms with percussion ignition. He also established a vinegar facility, where his distillation apparatus produced a popular alcoholic drink[35]. His interest in chemistry led him to set up a laboratory on his property, from which he sent papers to journals on producing sugar from potato starch and purifying turpentine. He came across chloroform in July 1831, arguably slightly before the other contenders, while attempting to produce a pesticide by distilling chlorinated lime and whiskey[vii]. It became popular with his neighbors as an intoxicating beverage which they called 'Guthrie's sweet whiskey.' Guthrie was not certain of its chemical structure, and wasn't aware that he had synthesized a new molecule instead of the 'chloric ether' which had been his goal, but he believed it had possibilities for other uses. It has been said that his 8-year-old daughter accidentally drank some and briefly fell into a deep sleep[36]. An alternative tale has it that a bottle was left open in his room and he became intoxicated and realized the medical implications. Guthrie began employing it as an inhaled anesthetic while performing amputations. Though he discussed his work with physicians in New Haven, they did not share his enthusiasm. In the next year or two, Guthrie, perhaps dispirited by the 100 or so explosions in his laboratory, seemed to lose his keenness for inventions. Instead, he turned his energy to his various commercial enterprises. Ultimately, the port of Sackett's Harbor, and his finances, languished with the decrease in boat traffic after the advent

---

[vii] Guthrie was working on a better way to synthesize 'chloric ether' (also known as 'Dutch oil' or 'Dutch liquid'), which apparently had been used as a solvent and pesticide, and had also been mentioned in the 1831 textbook *Elements of Chemistry* by Prof. Benjamin Stillman of Yale as a possible stimulant. Although Guthrie believed he had made Dutch liquid, which is thought to be the related compound dichlorethane, he had instead produced chloroform. For composition of Dutch liquid, see A. Faulconer and Keys, *Foundations of Anesthesiology*, Vol 1, p442, also cited in https://www.atticusrarebooks.com/pages/books/212/samuel-guthrie/new-mode-of-preparing-a-spirituous-solution-of-chloric-ether-in-american-journal-of-science-and-the. The Dutch liquid was originally prepared in the late 18th century by combining ethylene (Chapter Three) with chlorine.

of railway service to the area. Though he also had to deal with the death of one son and the debts of another, he is said to have maintained a positive outlook about the future until he passed away in October 1848[37].

Sixteen years after Guthrie's attempt to make a pesticide, chloroform found a champion in the Scottish obstetrician James Young Simpson (1811-1870). A baker's son, his abilities became evident at a young age, as he entered the University of Edinburgh at age fourteen and began studying medicine at sixteen. As a student, he witnessed Robert Liston, a noted surgeon, perform a mastectomy. Liston was a leading proponent of the view that the danger in surgery is directly proportional to its duration, and he was known for his speed. He was reputed to be able to perform a limb amputation in less than 30 seconds. Nonetheless, the agony of the awake but restrained woman was so startling to him that he left the room hurriedly and began to think of changing to the study of law. He ultimately decided to continue with medicine and dedicated himself to finding a method of relieving pain during surgery.

After becoming a professor of medicine and midwifery at the University of Edinburgh at age twenty-eight, Simpson continued to look for ways of easing pain in childbirth, including mesmerism. He learned about ether anesthesia in London in 1846 and began administering it during deliveries. Though effective, it had many drawbacks. It was an irritant to the respiratory system and often resulted in vomiting and other distress afterwards. Because it was very volatile, it often filled the room with vapor which could affect the staff, and it was also easily ignited and explosive. Although effective for brief dental procedures, he felt it was less applicable for prolonged surgery or childbirth. Simpson began looking for alternatives. He and two colleagues, Mathew Duncan and George Keith, had sessions of inhaling various possible chemical candidates, without success. Their notoriety was such that Simpson's neighbor, Prof. James Miller, was known to stop by in the mornings 'just to inquire if everyone was still alive.'[38]

In October 1847, David Waldie, a physician and chemist in the Liverpool Apothecaries Company who was visiting Scotland, mentioned that he provided it to doctors as an inhaled treatment for asthma and noted that some patients using it fell asleep. By some accounts, Waldie and one of his employers had experimented with chloroform on themselves, and Waldie recommended it to Simpson as a possible anesthetic[39].

Simpson pursued this lead with vigor. He recruited his long-suffering colleagues and met in his dining room at home. Watched over by his wife Jessie, they poured three tumblers of chloroform, which they inhaled and sipped. Simpson became intoxicated, and the other two, after a brief period of stimulation, fell asleep. Simson and one colleague ended up unconscious on the floor, the other apparently snoring loudly with his head on the table. Encouraged by the result, he later convinced his niece to smell the chloroform. She became giddy, then fell asleep after confusedly mumbling, 'I am an angel.'

It was not long before Simpson tried administering chloroform during childbirth, his patient being the daughter of another physician. He poured half a teaspoon onto a handkerchief, which he then shaped into a funnel, and placed it over her nose and mouth. Soon thereafter she gave birth, reporting that she had been unconscious and experienced no pain. She and her husband were so impressed that the baby was named Anesthesia. Years later, Simpson was given a picture of Anesthesia as a young woman, which was given a place of honor in his office.

Simpson described his results with a series of patients at a meeting of the medical society in Edinburgh in 1847. At the end of the talk, he passed around a silk handkerchief containing chloroform. Some of his colleagues became intoxicated and excited, much to the amusement of the others, while some fell unconscious. Many found the experience pleasant, and, overall, the response was enthusiastic. Chloroform became increasingly popular, though it had shaky beginnings. Compared to ether, it required greater care in administration to avoid often-fatal abnormal heart rhythms (ventricular fibrillation) or respiratory arrest, and it could result in severe liver damage.

Some women when first inhaling it became sexually aroused, bringing down condemnation in those Victorian times. There were religious concerns as well, which Simpson had faced since had had begun using ether. It was charged that God had intended childbirth to be painful, a view supported by Genesis 3:16. This view had been held for centuries, and indeed there had been a case in 1591 in which a Lady Eufame Macalyene had been denounced to the authorities in Edinburgh for requesting something to decrease the pain in childbirth, and as punishment she was burned at the stake. Simpson argued that the Bible could be interpreted to take a very different view, citing Genesis 2:21, in which God made Adam sleep while one of his ribs was removed and his flesh healed, resulting in Eve's creation. Chloroform's reputation also suffered as a result of its nefarious misuse in robberies and rapes.

Ultimately, the popularity of the medical use of chloroform was greatly increased by the work of John Snow (1813-1858). The son a coal yard laborer in York, he became a surgeon's apprentice at age fourteen and started medical school in London at age twenty-three. As a young doctor, he was very interested in cholera, which was then thought to result from tainted air, but which he believed to infect by an oral route. When there was an outbreak of cholera in Soho in 1854, he found that the only places in the area which seemed relatively disease-free were a brewery and an almshouse, which shared one thing—they did not obtain their water from a public pump on Broad Street. He convinced the authorities to remove the handle of the pump, which was a major source of water for the area, and the cases of cholera rapidly declined. This finding has led to his reputation of one of the earliest practitioners of medical epidemiology.

Snow was also very interested in anesthesia and collaborated with surgeons by administering ether and later chloroform. His success continued as he refined the methods and dosage in a systematic manner. In 1853, he was asked to give chloroform to Queen Victoria during the birth of her eighth child, Prince Leopold. Her praise of the experience, which she repeated two years later when Princess Beatrice was born, led to a rapid increase in its acceptance and popularity.[viii] Snow ultimately administered chloroform about 4,000 times without a fatality. In the late 1850s, his review of the world's literature described fifty deaths over a period of seven years.

[viii] This was but one of many examples of her remarkable influence of public opinion. Nine years later, for instance, when a company offering the first synthetic fabric dye was floundering, she wore a dress colored with the new 'aniline purple' to the Great Exhibition of 1862, and it rapidly became popular. As a result, the synthetic dye industry flourished, and later branched out into making paints, food coloring, fertilizers, and medicines. (For further information, please see *Molecules, Madness, and Malaria*, listed in the Selected Bibliography.)

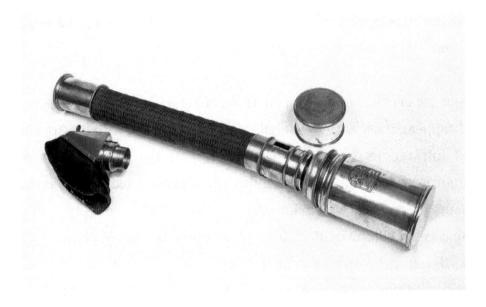

Figure 2-6: John Snow's chloroform inhaler.

Simpson went on to a fruitful career in which he developed the use of iron sutures, designed a new type of obstetric forceps, developed techniques of medical statistics, and wrote extensively on medical history. He seems to have had mixed feelings about his work with chloroform, which brought him fame. On the one hand, when he was chosen to write about anesthesia for the *Encyclopedia Britannica*, he requested that it be placed in the 'C' volume under 'Chloroform' and de-emphasized the histories of nitrous oxide and ether. Alternatively, he later felt some chagrin that many of these later achievements were overlooked in the widespread adulation of his work with chloroform. He died at his home on Queen Street, Edinburgh, at age fifty-eight. His family was offered a burial place in Westminster Abbey, but they chose instead to place him nearby in Edinburgh. Such was his renown that Scotland closed the stock market, banks, and businesses on the day of his funeral, and huge crowds watched the procession to the cemetery.

The use of chloroform as an anesthetic later declined and ultimately disappeared across the first half of the 20th century, with the advent of intravenous hexobarbital in 1932, and the development of improved gas anesthesia methods using nitrous oxide and, later, safer agents such as halothane in 1956. Studies also appeared suggesting carcinogenicity in mice. At one time, its sweet taste and analgesic properties led to it being used in small amounts in remedies for toothache as well as mouthwash, but this was eliminated in the U.S. in 1976. In more recent years, it has been mostly used as a chemical building block in the preparation of refrigerants, though this is being phased out. Chloroform can be spontaneously formed in chlorinated drinking water when the chlorine interacts with organic molecules, and the amount present is monitored by municipal agencies and is required to be below levels set by the Environmental Protection Agency.

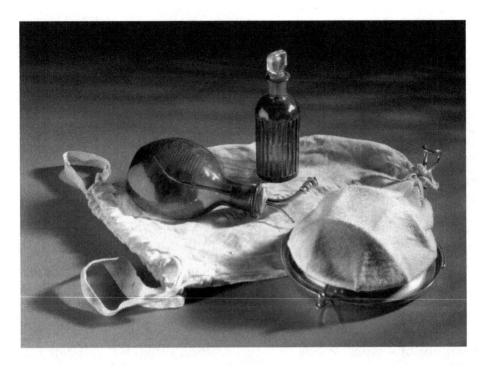

Figure 2-7: *Anesthetic kit, 1914-1918. It was designed for portability for use by the German army during World War I. Note the calibrations on the bottle to measure the amount of ether or chloroform to apply to the cotton cover stretched over the metal mask frame.*

<u>Non-medical use of chloroform:</u> We had mentioned earlier that part of the difficulty in acceptance of chloroform in the 1850s was its somewhat sinister reputation from criminal use in robberies and rapes. Perhaps the most notorious of these was a few decades later, in the case of Jack the Ripper, who some believe incapacitated or killed his victims with chloroform before performing his grisly deeds. Lest one have the impression that chloroform crimes are only the stuff of novels and movies set in Victorian alleyways, it should be noted that they still occasionally occur. In 1993, Samson Dubria, a San Diego physician, was

convicted of the murder of 20-year-old Jennifer Klapper, who had been found dead in a motel room, with evidence of chloroform poisoning. The jury did not accept Dr. Dubria's argument that she may have become affected by chloroform when they were driving behind a chemical truck, and he was given a life sentence. In 2014, Roger Cooper, a Costco manager in Coventry, England, and his brother David were convicted of killing 34-year-old Sameena Imam with chloroform which they had purchased online, apparently because he did not want his partner to find out about their affair. Both brothers received 30-year sentences before consideration of parole. In a 2018 case which has not yet been fully resolved, Mariah Kay Woods, a 3-year-old girl in North Carolina, was found at the bottom of a creek, inside a couch cushion weighted with cement. The autopsy reported that she had died of chloroform poisoning, and her mother's boyfriend was charged with murder. Though chloroform has long since been abandoned by the clinical medical profession, the idea of its illicit use, perhaps fueled by movies and literature, sadly still lingers on.

Synthetic hypnotics: Chloral hydrate and the road to the barbiturates

Choral hydrate, the first synthetic sleeping pill: In the 1860s, there was increased interest in new sedative agents. Some have speculated that this resulted from the popularity of ether and chloroform, while others have noted that the increase in patients in mental asylums in Europe and the U.S. during the decade may have emphasized the need for new medicines. Chloral hydrate had been synthesized by the German chemist Justus von Liebig in 1832 in the process of chlorinating ethanol, not long after he had made chloroform in 1831. Its sleep-inducing properties were not fully appreciated until 1869, when the German pharmacologist Otto Liebreich (1839-1908), following on the work of Rudolf Buchheim (1820-1879), demonstrated its clinical effects on medical inpatients, as well as psychiatric patients, at Berlin's Charité Asylum. In addition to sedation, he believed that it ameliorated delirium tremens and might be useful in other situations as well. Soon European journals were publishing a variety of supportive studies. The prominent Austrian psychiatrist Richard von Krafft-Ebing, known for his work in sexual psychopathology and other areas, pronounced it helpful in psychoneurosis.

Both Liebreich and Buchheim were mistaken in their understanding of the chemistry of chloral hydrate, believing it to be converted in the body to chloroform, while it was later learned that it is metabolized to trichloroethanol (chloral). A mistake in the theory of its chemistry did not limit its effectiveness, however, and after millennia in which plant-based potions were the only source of sedatives, the first fully synthetic sedative and sleeping medicine became available. It was one of the early steps in the evolution of organic chemistry, which had its roots in the synthesis of urea in 1828, and later it was accelerated with the founding of the synthetic dye industry in 1856. These newfound skills in turn evolved into making many other kinds of products, including medicines[40].

Although the use of chloral hydrate initially was oriented toward asylum patients, it rapidly became popular as a sedative and sleep medicine in the general community. As a synthetic substance, its dosing could be much more precise than that of plant-based substances such as morphine, and, unlike morphine, it did not require injections. Its limitations also began to appear. It was dependence-producing, and abrupt discontinuation of high doses could result in a life-threatening withdrawal syndrome. By the late 19th century, it became a drug of abuse for a number of well-known personages.

Among those who suffered from chloral hydrate abuse was the London poet and painter Dante Gabriel Rossetti (1828-1882), a leader of the Pre-Raphaelites, who revolted against Victorian painting techniques and emphasized a return to the intense colors and detail of Italian art before the Renaissance. Originally highlighting a return to nature, they turned their attention in the 1850s to a romanticized version of Arthurian legends and medieval times. Their muse was a beautiful but troubled young woman named Elizabeth Siddall, who married Rossetti, later dying of an overdose of opium in 1862. As an expression of his grief, Rossetti buried his unpublished poems with her in London's Highgate Cemetery.

As time went on, Rossetti's paintings tended to downplay medieval themes, and more often portrayed conventionally beautiful women. He became more interested in his poetry. Recalling the popularity of his translation of Italian poems some years before, in 1869, he began to wonder whether publication of his earlier poems might be a successful endeavor. He was convinced by Charles Augustus Howell, a shady art dealer and likely blackmailer[ix], to allow him to open his wife's casket and remove the poems, which were quickly published with some fanfare. What Rossetti didn't anticipate was that they were harshly criticized by a critic named Robert Buchanan, who objected to their sensuous nature. Upset, Rossetti published an imprudent rebuttal, which only led to more and more publicity about their animosity.

Rossetti also developed trouble sleeping, and in 1969, the year chloral hydrate became available, he learned about it from a friend who was an American journalist. He began taking it in higher and higher amounts, often in combination with alcohol to disguise the taste or increase the rapidity of effect. After 1872, he became more of a recluse, and though he continued to paint and write, his deterioration became evident in hallucinations and delusions of persecution. A stroke and likely kidney disease contributed to his decline, and in 1882, he passed away at a friend's home. His final wish was to not be laid to rest in Highgate Cemetery.

Many other historical figures turned out to suffer from overuse of chloral hydrate. As described in *The curious history of medicines in*

[ix] Howell's nefarious activities were said to be the basis for the Sherlock Holmes story by Arthur Conan Doyle entitled *The Adventure of Charles Augustus Milverton*.

psychiatry[41], after Abraham Lincoln's death, his wife Mary Todd Lincoln received high doses from her doctors, which may have contributed to her later delusions and hallucinations and admission to an asylum. Chloral hydrate also developed a kind of notoriety for being the main constituent of the 'Mickey Finn,' a drink named after a Chicago bartender who was tried in 1903 for drugging his customers. According to one of the bar girls, 'Gold Tooth' Mary Thornton, he then robbed them and placed them in an alley to awaken the next morning with little memory of what happened.

Abuse of chloral hydrate declined as the 20th century progressed, though it continued to appear, occasionally in some startling cases. In 1952, for instance, the country singer Hank Williams came under the influence of 'Doctor' Toby Marshall, a forger and ex-convict who had purchased a diploma for $25, and plied him with chloral hydrate and other drugs. After having consumed chloral hydrate and alcohol, and having pre-existing heart disease, he died in 1953 late at night in a car on the way to a concert in Ohio.

The medical use of chloral hydrate also declined with the recognition of its hazards, as well as the advent of newer sleeping medicines, but it is still on the market. It is little used, aside from sedation for pediatric diagnostic procedures and surgery, and this too is now rare.

Barbituric acid: The story of the cyclic compound barbituric acid, which later became the basis for the clinically used barbiturate sedatives, hypnotics, and anesthetics in the 20th century, begins with the German chemist Adolph von Bayer (1835-1917). The son of a Prussian general, he began chemical experiments at home when nine years old, and within a few years had created a formerly unknown copper compound. After undergraduate work and time in the army, he went to the University of Heidelberg to study chemistry under Robert Bunsen. After a quarrel, he came to work with August Kekulé, who was pioneering an understanding of the manner in which carbon atoms bind to each other, and was to go on to envision how they might form ring-like compounds. (For a detailed description of Kekulé and his work, please see *Molecules, Madness, and Malaria*[42].) After getting his graduate degree, he followed Kekulé to Ghent, Belgium. There, Kekulé assigned him to the task of making a cyclic molecule out of two unlikely components, malonic acid (derived from apples) and urea, found in urine.

Happily, von Bayer was successful in 1864, and he marked the occasion by going to a tavern. When he arrived, however, a celebration was already under way. Soldiers from the nearby barracks were commemorating the day of Saint Barbara, the patron saint of the artillery. During the alcohol-fueled celebration, it is thought that the words 'Barbara' and 'urea' were somehow combined into the word 'barbiturate' to describe the new chemical compound. Stories differ in this regard, some involving a barmaid named Barbara who may have supplied specimens to the chemical project. Others argue that the name came from the German word *schlusselbart*, part of a key, as he foresaw that it might be the key to many related compounds. As time went on, perhaps 2,500 barbiturates were made, of which about 50 became clinically used medicines

Von Bayer went on to make a number of other important discoveries. Along with a colleague, Heinrich Caro, he synthesized indigo dye, which had intrigued him ever since he bought a sample to study at age thirteen. Historically one of the first dyes employed for fabrics and printing (and now well known for the color of blue jeans), indigo had previously been available primarily from plants found in India. It was now possible to create it in the laboratory, and with later refinements by others, in industrial quantities. Von Bayer also developed fluorescent dyes, as well as a building block for what later became the first plastic, Bakelite. For these discoveries, he received the Nobel Prize in 1905.

CHAPTER THREE: THE BARBITURATES AND INHALATIONAL ANESTHETICS THROUGH HALOTHANE (EARLY TO MID-20th CENTURY)

The barbiturate sedatives: A vacation in Verona

Although the barbituric acid discovered by von Bayer was a crucial achievement, it did not itself cause sedation. It was not until 1903 that barbital, the first barbiturate with sedative properties, was developed. The story began with Joseph von Mering (1849-1908), a German physician who, along with Oscar Minkowski, had previously discovered that the pancreas secreted a substance which regulates blood sugar, later identified as insulin. Von Mering was now interested in sedatives. He noted that in another older group of drugs known as sulfonals, modification by including ethyl groups (two carbon atoms linked together and associated hydrogen atoms) enhanced their soporific qualities. He wondered if this idea might be applied to urea derivatives, and to this end joined with Emil Fischer (1852-1919), a former student of von Bayer and a famous chemist in his own right. The two worked on combining diethyl malonic acid with urea. When the resultant compound, barbital, was found to potently sedate animals, von Mering telegraphed the good news to

Fischer, who was on vacation in Italy. Fischer's response was that a good trade name for the new drug might be Veronal, named after Verona, which he considered to be a remarkably restful place. (Another version of the story is that he named it after *vera*, the Latin word for 'true,' as he thought it the first true hypnotic.) Veronal was to become the most commonly prescribed barbiturate until the advent of phenobarbital in 1912.

As for Fischer and von Mering, both received Nobel prizes, in 1902 and 1901, respectively. Fischer had had a remarkable career in which he discovered hydrazine (later used as rocket fuel and, surprisingly, as a building block for the first antidepressants [43]) and made advances in understanding the chemistry of sugars and purines, which were later found to be among the building blocks of DNA. Von Mering, as we mentioned earlier, along with his colleague Oskar Minkowski, had made the first observations that the pancreas releases a substance later identified as insulin.

Intravenous barbiturates for anesthesia: Although barbital and phenobarbital were very effective for many uses, including as daytime sedatives and anticonvulsants, they were relatively long-acting drugs and not suitable for anesthesia. As time went on, the more rapid-acting hexobarbital, which could be given intravenously, was marketed as Evipan by the Bayer company in 1932 and became popular as an agent to induce anesthesia. It continued to be employed through the 1940s and 1950s, though declining after the advent by others such as thiopental (sodium thiopental, sodium pentothal), whose very short duration of action made adjustments of depth of anesthesia easier. Its limitations were that, like all barbiturates, it was less effective for muscle relaxation and did not by itself provide relief from pain. Hexobarbital was a turning point in anesthesia, in that it marked the beginning of the decline of chloroform. It also paved the way for later intravenous anesthetics including ketamine, etomidate, midazolam, and propofol.

Though useful as an induction agent, there was a long road in learning to use it and other barbiturates safely. It was alleged at one point that thiopental, which as we noted largely replaced hexobarbital, may have contributed in its early years to a number of surgical deaths during emergency treatment of the wounded from Pearl Harbor, though the degree to which this occurred was later questioned. More experience was gained, and it was in wide use until the advent of the intravenous agent propofol, which is now the most common induction agent. It is now rarely used partly from issues of supply and also its past association with legal executions.

Non-medical use of barbiturates: Just as the euphoriant qualities of earlier agents led to sharing nitrous oxide at social events, and the advent of 'ether frolics,' it did not take long for the abuse potential of barbiturates to become evident. Repeated use leads to tolerance (progressive decrease in effects leading to taking higher doses). The Russian tsarina Alexandra Feodorovna found this to be the case, complaining that 'I'm literally saturated with it.'[44] Sudden cessation from large doses could lead to an often-fatal withdrawal syndrome with tremors, hallucinations, very high temperatures, seizures, and other symptoms. They were widely misused as oral 'downers' in the 1950s and 1960s as exemplified in Jacqueline Susann's blockbuster 1966 novel *Valley of the Dolls*[45], portraying three ambitious young women whose lives were complicated by their frequent misuse of stimulants and 'dolls' (barbiturates). This was most vividly seen in Frank Robson's 1967 movie version, in which Sharon Tate (1943-1969) played Jennifer North, a chorus dancer from New York who became involved in the fast life in Hollywood, but ultimately along with her friends came to a bad end. Barbiturates also frequently appeared in lethal overdoses, including well-publicized ones of famous figures including Marilyn Monroe, Elvis Presley, Judy Garland, Charles Boyer, Jimi Hendrix, and many others.

From the earliest days after the advent of hexobarbital, it and later barbiturates also took on a sinister air due to purposeful poisonings, both in fiction and in fact. A lethal combination of Evipan and Veronal appears, for instance in *Cards on the Table*, a 1937 Agatha Christie story. Sadly, in real life, the Nazis used hexobarbital for executing prisoners in concentration camps[46]. Thiopental for some time was part of the lethal cocktail used in legal executions in the U.S. It has not been used for this purpose since 2011, after authorities in Italy, where it was being made, passed a ruling banning its use in executions. A broader ban on drugs for capital punishment was also passed by the European Union in 2011. During the time of writing this book, on the week of July 13, 2020, the U.S. federal government executed three death row prisoners, the first in seventeen years, with intravenous pentobarbital given alone[47] and obtained from sources which the government had kept confidential[48].

Historically, thiopental and other drugs such as sodium amytal, scopolamine, and midazolam have also been misused by intelligence agencies or law enforcement agencies as a 'truth serum' in an effort to make prisoners less resistant to withholding information. One famous example was in the follow-up to the Kennedy assassination, in which the District Attorney of New Orleans ordered a thiopental interview of Perry Russo, an acquaintance of David Ferrie, who was speculated to be part of the plot. In general, the courts have ruled that information gained in this way is invalid, and many psychiatrists have argued that subjects under such drugs are very suggestible. It seems likely that these drugs make a person more voluble in providing information, regardless of its accuracy or lack thereof.

Early inhalational anesthetics after chloroform

Ethylene and the mystery of the wilting carnations: In 1908, workers at the Hull Botanical Laboratory, affiliated with the University of Chicago, noticed that something in the burning gas which was used for lighting caused carnations and other flowers to close. Although it was originally thought that this might be due to carbon monoxide, it turned out to be a consequence of ethylene, which comprised four percent of illuminating gas, and which also was an industrial chemical used in welding. Some years later, Arno Luckhardt and J. Bailey Carter at the University of Chicago explored its biological effects further. At first, they thought it might combine with hemoglobin in the same manner as carbon monoxide, with lethal consequences, but this turned out not to be the case. Frogs and rats exposed to an ethylene/oxygen mixture became stuporous, but they awakened quickly and without obvious ill effects when they were placed back in room air. This led the investigators to wonder whether it might be useful as a human anesthetic. After elaborate animal studies, Luckhardt and Bailey breathed an ethylene/oxygen mixture themselves until unconsciousness. In order to determine its safety, Luckhardt did so another 700 times in amounts approaching anesthesia before being fully convinced. They then made it available to Presbyterian Hospital in Chicago. In 1923, they presented data on 106 patients who had had successful surgery with ethylene anesthesia. After there had been experience with some 900 cases, they made it available for general use without patenting it, a remarkable contrast to the struggles for private gain after the discovery of ether (Chapter Two).

Ethylene is a simple organic molecule comprised of two linked carbon atoms, associated with four hydrogen atoms. [x] It was

---

[x] Ethylene got its name from a 19th century practice of adding a Greek female suffix to molecules which are formed by removing one hydrogen atom from the parent compound. Thus ethylene ('daughter of ethyl') with the formula C_2H_4 was derived from ethyl (C_2H_5).

originally made by slowly exposing small amounts of ethyl alcohol to heated sulfuric or orthophosphoric acids. It turned out that it had been known to Dutch chemists in the late 18th century and was one of the components of 'Dutch liquid,' which Samuel Guthrie was trying to produce more efficiently in 1831 when he stumbled upon chloroform. Ethylene was first synthesized in 1779 by the Dutch physician and scientist Jan Ingenhauss (1730-1799), a correspondent with Benjamin Franklin, and its soporific effect in animals had been described as early as 1885. In humans, its benefits appeared to be that induction was swift, with no irritation to the respiratory system, and there appeared to be less discoloration of the skin due to low oxygen levels ('cyanosis') than with previous agents. Recovery was rapid, with minimal nausea and vomiting. In the late 1920s, it was seen as a contender to replace nitrous oxide.

One concern about the use of ethylene was that muscle relaxation was not always adequate, especially for abdominal surgery, which often required supplemental ether. Another was its strong odor. The most serious problem was its explosiveness, a hazard in operating rooms where cautery or other electrical equipment was being used. For these reasons, by the 1940s, it gradually began to go out of favor and was replaced by safer agents.

Before we leave the topic of ethylene, we should come back to the unhappy fate of the carnations in the Hull Botanical Laboratory in 1908. It turns out that ethylene is also a natural plant hormone with many regulatory functions, including promoting flower senescence [49]. It is still used commercially for ripening and enhancing color in tomatoes, citrus, pears, bananas, and other fruit.

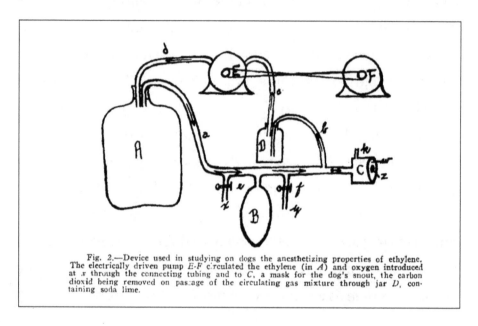

Fig. 2.—Device used in studying on dogs the anesthetizing properties of ethylene. The electrically driven pump E-F circulated the ethylene (in A) and oxygen introduced at x through the connecting tubing and to C, a mask for the dog's snout, the carbon dioxid being removed on passage of the circulating gas mixture through jar D, containing soda lime.

Figure 3-1: Apparatus used by Arno Luckhardt and J.B. Carter to study the effects of ethylene and oxygen on dogs, 1923. Ethylene is supplied from the bottle 'A', oxygen from a hose 'x', and circulated by use of a pump and motor ('E' and 'F'). A bottle of soda lime ('D') is used to absorb carbon dioxide. The animal would breathe through the mask 'C' on the right side.

Cyclopropane: The substance itself, comprised of a ring structure of three carbon atoms, each attached to two hydrogen atoms, was first made in 1881 by August Freund, an Austrian academic chemist in what is now western Ukraine. There were no significant uses for it until its anesthetic qualities were recognized in the late 1920s and early 1930s. Its clinical application largely began with Ralph Waters (1883-1979), an American physician at the

University of Wisconsin who had an important role in developing anesthesia as a medical specialty. He administered the non-irritating gas with a petroleum odor using a closed system in which excess carbon dioxide was absorbed (again something he was key in developing), largely because of expense.

Though a potent anesthetic, cyclopropane also had many limitations. Partly because the ring was comprised of only three carbon atoms, there was considerable strain on its structure, contributing to making it highly flammable. Upon recovering from anesthesia, patients also tended to have disastrous drops in blood pressure and abnormal heart rhythms, which came to be known as 'cyclopropane shock.' This, in combination with the hazards of manufacturing and using it, led to its decline. Later, it tended to be employed only for induction of anesthesia, and it disappeared clinically in the 1980s.[xi]

Trichloroethylene— How a metal de-greaser became an anesthetic: First made in 1864 by the German chemist Emil Fischer (1852-1919), who also had a role in developing the first clinically used barbiturate (see Chapter Two), trichloroethylene was used as a solvent and for cleaning grease from metal. It was found that some people who used it developed loss of sensation in parts of

---

[xi] Cyclopropane is mostly of interest because it and nitrous oxide were among the earliest instances of anesthetics whose mechanism of action included inhibiting NMDA receptors in the nervous system, which took on more importance after the later development of the intravenous anesthetic ketamine (see later in this chapter).

the face and mouth which are served by the trigeminal nerve. As it happens, there is a condition known as trigeminal neuralgia, in which a malfunction of the nerve leads to pain in these areas, and by 1915, doctors were using this side effect of trichloroethylene as a treatment. By the late 1920s and early 1930s, it was noted that some patients receiving it became unconscious, and interest grew in using it as a possible anesthetic in the mid-1930s. The British, facing the likelihood of war, were eager to have less-flammable anesthetics, and ultimately it was manufactured by Imperial Chemical Industries, who later made halothane (Chapter Three). It was also initially perceived to have the advantage of not damaging the liver, and it lacked the pungent odor of ether.

Trichloroethylene did not have ideal properties, and indeed was less successful at creating states of deep anesthesia. It had low volatility, that is, it did not evaporate easily, and was greatly absorbed into tissues, making it slower in inducing anesthesia. It could be irritating to the airway as well as the eyes and skin, and though much less flammable than ether, could burn if exposed to high temperatures. Its decomposition products turned out to be toxic. By 1944, there were reports of surgical patients who had received it developing cranial nerve palsies. This effect was so potent that even patients who had been given other anesthetics developed nerve conditions apparently due to tiny amounts of decomposition products of trichloroethylene left over in the anesthesia machinery. It could cause very rapid breathing ('tachypnea') and heart arrhythmias, and contrary to early impressions, could result in liver damage. Though it remained in use in some areas as a self-administered anesthesia during childbirth, its popularity declined rapidly after the development of halothane in 1956.

Trichloroethylene was also used as an ingredient in some glues (which were sometimes abused by sniffing for the euphoriant effect), in cosmetics, and as a solvent in making decaffeinated coffee. With the growing evidence of toxicity as well as possible fetal damage and carcinogenicity, the U.S. Food and Drug Administration banned these practices in 1977, and its medical use disappeared in developed countries in the 1980s. It remains an industrial chemical for making refrigerants and degreasing equipment, and there have been a number of lawsuits about the public health consequences of its seepage into groundwater.

Xenon

Xenon is an inert gas which makes up a small fraction of the atmosphere (perhaps one part in 11.5 million) and is extracted during the process of fractionating air into oxygen and nitrogen. It was originally discovered, along with krypton and neon, by William Ramsay and Morris Travers, Scottish and English chemists, respectively, in the late 1890s, while evaporating liquid air. In modern times, xenon has a wide range of uses, including in lasers and flash lamps used in photography, medical imaging, and in ion propulsion engines in spacecraft.

In the late 1940s, there were reports that xenon-oxygen mixtures had soporific effects on mice, and by 1951 these observations had been extended to humans. This led to its development as an anesthetic, for which it has a number of desirable qualities. Because it is minimally soluble in blood and tissues, induction and awakening are relatively rapid. It has potent analgesic effects, more than nitrous oxide, which is the only other inhaled anesthetic with significant pain-reducing qualities. It produces minimal depression of cardiovascular function. It also offers some protection to the nervous system and cardiovascular system from injury due to lack of oxygen. It may have a relatively high rate of post-operative nausea and vomiting compared to other inhaled anesthetics, however.

The mechanism by which xenon produces anesthesia is not fully understood but involves, in part, being an antagonist at NMDA receptors (see ketamine section in Chapter Four), and this may also play a role in how it has nervous system protective qualities. Probably because of cost, there is no significant recreational abuse of xenon. In the early 2000s, there were some reports of doping of Russian athletes to improve performance, which was based on some data that it might indirectly increase the amount of red blood cells. The World Anti-Doping Agency prohibited this use of xenon in 2014.

Due to its relatively high cost, as well as scarcity of the devices for administering and recycling it, xenon has been used less in clinical anesthesia, and primarily in Europe. With the growing recognition of environmental issues, there has been more awareness that nitrous oxide may help deplete ozone in the atmosphere, and that there may be advantages to replacing it with xenon, which is not a greenhouse gas. Newer improvements in methods of administration and recycling have led to less xenon being needed for procedures, and there is growing interest in using it for anesthesia.

Halothane: How atomic bomb research led to the halogenated inhalational anesthetics

Halothane and later inhaled anesthetics can in a sense be considered derivatives of ether.[50] Adding halogen atoms (fluorine, chlorine, bromine, and others) to hydrocarbons in general produces greater anesthetic potency and reduces flammability. Halothane was discovered by Charles Walter Suckling (1920-2013), a chemist at Imperial Chemical Industries, in an effort to find anesthetics without the drawbacks of ether, chloroform, and trichloroethylene. During World War II, he had had experience with halogenated compounds, which were used among other things in making aviation fuel and enriching uranium.[xii,51] Indeed, he had been part of the 'Tube Alloys' group in Merseyside, a cover organization for Britain's contribution to making the atomic bomb. The knowledge gained in this research was important in the subsequent development of halogenated inhaled anesthetics.

[xii] In order to enrich uranium currently, the 'yellowcake' ore (uranium oxide powder) is combined with fluorine to produce uranium hexafluoride gas, which is then centrifuged to separate out the uranium-235. The enriched material is then converted to a powder of uranium dioxide, which is pressed into pellets.

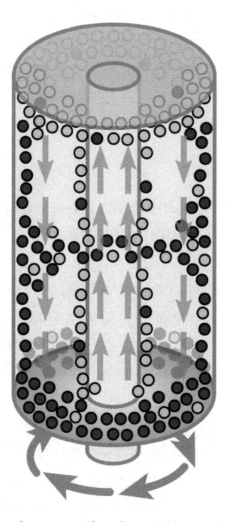

Figure 3-2: Diagram of a gas centrifuge for enriching uranium. As described in footnote xii, uranium ore is combined with fluorine to produce a gas which is a mixture of U235 (light blue) and the heavier U238 (dark blue). In the process of spinning, the two are separated so that U238 moves to the outer edges, then with heating, the U235 moves to the top, where it is collected. Knowledge of halogen chemistry gained through atomic research is thought to have been important to the later development of halogenated anesthetics. An offshoot of the Manhattan Project and the Malinkrodt company unsuccessfully pursued research in fluorinated anesthetics, but Charles Suckling, who had worked in Britain's atomic research during the war, succeeded with the synthesis of halothane in 1951.

In working on a new anesthetic, Suckling knew that adding halogen atoms decreased flammability, and that adding fluorine atoms in particular lowered the boiling point so that there was sufficient volatility. It also turned out that the presence of at least one hydrogen atom was required for the compound to have anesthetic properties.[52] With these thoughts in mind, in 1951, he synthesized halothane, which contains the halogens fluorine, chlorine, and bromine attached to carbon atoms, and after preliminary tests in mealworms and houseflies, turned it over to pharmacologists to study in animals. Samples were supplied to anesthesiologists at Oxford's Nuffield Department of Anesthetics, who first tested it on themselves. (Indeed there was a long history of doing so: in 1943, Dr. Edgar Pask from the same department, while in the Royal Air Force, had volunteered to be anesthetized with ether until respiratory arrest in order to test various methods of resuscitation.) [xiii, 53] By 1956, halothane was being used clinically by Michael Johnstone, a Manchester anesthesiologist, and it was soon on the market.

Although a major step forward, and valuable because it was not explosive or irritating to the airway, and indeed could dilate the bronchi to some degree, halothane's limitations also became apparent. It was very soluble in blood and tissues, which in general

---

[xiii] On another occasion, the intrepid professor agreed to be anesthetized, then placed in a water tank at a movie studio which was equipped with a wave-making apparatus, in order to test the Mae West life jackets designed to keep afloat unconscious pilots who had crashed into the water.

is a quality leading to slower recovery. Higher doses could suppress respiration and induce abnormal heart rhythms. By the late 1950s, cases of liver damage (which came to be known as the potentially lethal 'halothane hepatitis') began to be recognized, and though occurring in only one in thousands of cases, may have been the impetus for searching for safer agents. It could also produce malignant hyperthermia, a condition causing not only high temperatures, but also metabolic disturbances, rapid heartbeat, and muscle rigidity. Its use declined with the advent of the newer inhalable anesthetics from the late 1970s through the 1990s, and it is no longer available in the U.S., though still found in some developing countries. Its importance lies in its role as a step toward newer agents such as isoflurane, desflurane, and sevoflurane.

Halothane was also an early example of what came to be known as rational drug design, the process of creating drugs by systematically manipulating molecules with a goal based on an understanding of its effects, or knowledge of physiology or disease processes.[54] Put in this context, the movement in anesthesia from drugs accidentally discovered (chloroform in 1831 or ethylene in 1923) to purposeful design of molecules (halothane in 1951) is similar to the same process in other fields. In psychiatry, for instance, through the 1950s and 1960s, drugs tended to be discovered by astute individuals making unexpected observations. Iproniazid, the first monoamine oxidase inhibitor antidepressant, for instance, was originally a tuberculosis drug, and doctors noted that there was an improvement in mood in patients who took it. Similarly, chlorpromazine

(Thorazine) came about because a surgeon who was using it in studies of surgical shock noted that patients developed a state of relaxed indifference and wondered if it might be useful in psychiatric patients. [55] In contrast, by the 1980s, the first selective serotonin reuptake blocker (SSRI) was clinically developed at Eli Lilly and Company by modifying molecules with a goal of increasing amounts of serotonin in light of a theory that this might aid in depression. [56] Coming back to anesthesia, then, the advent of halothane represented a movement into more systematic development inside pharmaceutical houses seen in other areas. Among the inhalational anesthetics developed later by this approach were isoflurane, desflurane, and sevoflurane, discussed in the postscript.

CHAPTER FOUR: INTRAVENOUS DRUGS FOR SLEEP AND ANESTHESIA: BENZODIAZEPINES, KETAMINE, ETOMIDATE, PROPOFOL, DEXMEDETOMIDINE (SECOND HALF OF THE 20th CENTURY)

Benzodiazepines (oral and intravenous): How discarded fabric dyes evolved into sedatives

Leo Sternbach (1908-2005) was a pharmacologist who trained and then taught in Poland at the University of Krakow. His Jewish heritage made it difficult to work at the university, and ultimately, he came to be employed by the Hoffman LaRoche pharmaceutical company in Switzerland. Facing the uncertainties after the German invasion of Greece and Yugoslavia in 1941, he settled in their new headquarters in New Jersey. He was known as brilliant in the laboratory, but his propensity for showing disdain for his superiors (reminiscent of Paracelsus, in Chapter One) led to frequent transfers. During those years, the company was a major source of vitamins for the allies. At one point, Sternbach discovered a new method of producing biotin (Vitamin B7), which was marketed and gave him more security while he continued to try and follow his own directions in research.

When the tranquilizer meprobamate, produced by a rival company, became extremely popular in 1953, he was asked to see if he could produce one for Hoffman LaRoche. Other companies were taking the time-honored approach of making small changes to the meprobamate molecule; instead, Sternbach was asked to find something completely new. He selected as his starting point a group of azo dyes he had worked on during his training, which had not been fruitful for this purpose but might be useful for building blocks in this new project. To this end, he produced about forty variations and passed them on to his colleagues for behavioral testing. None produced a profile suggesting tranquilization, and eventually his superiors decided to drop the project, and they asked him to move on to work on antibiotics.

A few years later, in 1957, one of his assistants, while cleaning the shelves, noticed an old, unused bottle, which evidently was the fortieth in the series of compounds from his previous work. He asked what he should do with it, and Sternbach, who had been directed to be working on something new, instead asked his colleagues to run it through the behavioral tests for tranquilizing. When they did so, it turned out to cause sedation and muscle relaxation. It appeared to decrease aggression, and later a well-known photo collage showed a forty-pound lynx with a fierce expression changed by the medicine into a gentle feline smelling a flower. There were comparable results in monkeys, baboons, kangaroos, and tigers. Human studies with high doses initially showed sedation, dizziness, and slurred speech. On one memorable occasion, Sternbach tested it on himself with this result, much to the alarm of his family (as had James Young Simpson with chloroform a century before). Later, with lower doses, patients manifested the reductions in anxiety with minimal sedation, which had been the goal

In 1960, the original compound chlordiazepoxide came to market as Librium (from 'equilibrium'), followed by Valium, and a decade later flurazepam (Dalmane), designated for sleep, and in 1975 midazolam (Versed), an intravenous anesthetic. The benzodiazepines became very widely used, partly because they were believed to be safer than barbiturates. Indeed, in some senses they were, particularly regarding single-drug overdoses (although when taken in combination with alcohol or other drugs they could be very toxic). In terms of sleep, they were thought to be advantageous in that they did not produce the marked suppression of REM sleep seen with the barbiturates. (As it turned out, however, they did produce a marked decrease in slow-wave sleep.) Over the years, their limitations became more apparent. They were dependence-producing and came to be listed by the Drug Enforcement Administration as Schedule IV agents. Studies revealed that many, particularly the longer-acting ones, could affect driving, and that they could cause confusional states in the elderly. Some studies associated their use with the later development of dementia, although others have questioned this. The FDA in 2016 required 'black box' warnings about the potentially lethal consequences of combining them with opiates. For these and other concerns, their use for anxiety has declined in favor of the SSRI antidepressants, and their administration for sleep was seen at least initially as less favorable with the advent of the 'Z drugs' (see postscript). Intravenous midazolam continues to be used for sedation preoperatively, for sedation and amnesia during medical procedures such as endoscopies, for intubated patients in the intensive care unit, and less commonly since the advent of propofol, for anesthesia induction.

Sternbach himself went on to other things, creating a variety of medicines and filing some 241 patents. He didn't benefit financially very much, making only $1 for each of the patent rights he assigned to the company. But his intent had been something else—to have freedom to let his research take him where they may, and indeed he made contributions involving minimizing bleeding during brain surgery and treating hypertension. Even after retiring in the early 1970s, he maintained an office at the company, coming to work most days until his mid-nineties.

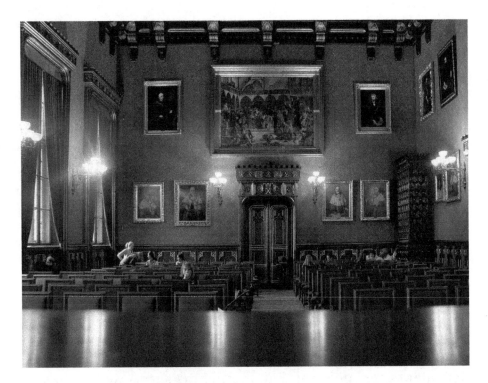

Figure 4-1: Lecture hall at the University of Krakow, 2015. Sternbach got his doctorate degree in organic chemistry there in 1931 and continued further training and teaching there for another five years. While a post-doctoral student, he worked on a group of azo dyes and related compounds (benzoheptoxodiazines), which were not found to be satisfactory for fabrics. Twenty years later, when searching for a chemical starting point for a new tranquilizer, he recalled these dyes, which ultimately were the building blocks for what became the benzodiazepines.

Ketamine

Ketamine in anesthesia: Ketamine was an outgrowth of research with phencyclidine, which was created in the 1950s by V. Harold Maddox, a medicinal chemist at the Parke Davis company. On the basis of animal studies, it was proposed as a possible anesthetic, but when used in humans it was found to produce significant post-surgery delirium, and in further testing it was confirmed to be a hallucinogen. Though PCP was clearly not acceptable as a clinical anesthetic[xiv], it was thought that the family from which it came might contain a medicine of interest. To this end, Calvin Lee Stevens at Wayne State University, who was affiliated with Parke Davis, created a number of variations on the phencyclidine molecule. In 1962, he produced ketamine, which was much less potent and appeared to have anesthetic properties in animals. It was first tested in humans in 1964 and approved for clinical use in the U.S. in 1970. The timing of its release was such that it was used widely during surgery in the Vietnam War.

Ketamine is very different than most of the agents we have talked about in that it produces dissociation, a sense of feeling detached from the world, which does not seem real, or depersonalization, a sense that one is an outside observer. While under the influence of the drug, a person appears sedated or even in a trance-like condition. There is decreased pain sensation and amnesia afterwards.

Some advantages of ketamine are that there is relatively good preservation of respiration, reflexes in the airway, and cardiac function. It is not an airway irritant and indeed has bronchodilating

---

[xiv] Phencyclidine (PCP) went on to become an illicit drug of abuse, with street names such as angel dust, love boat, rocket fuel, and others.

effects. It is approved as the sole anesthetic agent when muscle relaxation is not needed, as an induction agent followed by other anesthetics, to supplement relatively weaker agents such as nitrous oxide, or for sedation during uncomfortable procedures.

Because of emergence reactions, which appear in roughly 12 percent, and include hallucinations and delirium, its use in practice often tends to be in situations which take advantage of its rapidity and relatively small effects on blood pressure and respiration. Thus, it is sometimes given, for instance, in emergency rooms in trauma patients and in military medicine. In non-emergency practice, probably its most common use is in outpatient surgery in which a patient is not intubated. In this situation, it is often given in combination with a benzodiazepine to minimize hallucinations or other side effects. It is also used off-label for pain management, for instance, in trauma or post-operatively.

Ketamine in psychiatry: Since the 1990s, there has been interest in using low doses of intravenous ketamine as an antidepressant, particularly for patients who have not responded to traditional antidepressants. Infusions typically take about forty-five minutes and are often given in a series of six treatments during a roughly two-week period. Unlike most antidepressants, benefits in mood often appear very rapidly, often on the same day. Suicidal thoughts in particular seem to improve and are not necessarily related to general improvement in mood. The duration of the response varies and may be as short as a few days or extend for several weeks. In either event, this is much longer than the time ketamine remains in the body. This seems to indicate that the benefits result not so much from the actual presence of the drug, but rather from changes it makes in the nervous system. This is sometimes suggested to involve building new connections in neural pathways, though the specifics are not yet well understood. Some work in animals suggests that various forms of stress reduce the number of spines on the dendrites of neurons (part of the receiving apparatus in the connections between cells) in part of the brain's prefrontal cortex, and that these are replaced after ketamine treatment.[57]

Side effects of a single dose of ketamine given as an antidepressant include feeling strange or loopy or bizarre, as well as visual distortions; generally, these last less than four hours.[58] Over the course of treatment, rarely some patients may develop periods of hallucinations and confusion. Some people experience brief periods of increased blood pressure, or nausea and vomiting. Persons who use ketamine repeatedly for recreational purposes may develop irritation of the bladder ('ulcerative cystitis'), resulting in incontinence and sometimes blood in the urine.

Ketamine has so many different effects on the nervous system that it has sometimes been called a 'pharmacologist's nightmare.' One aspect involves blocking the function of the NMDA receptor, one of the types of receptors for glutamate, the major excitatory neurotransmitter in the nervous system.[xv]

Ketamine itself is not specifically approved by the FDA for depression, and hence has been used 'off-label.' In March 2019, however, approval was given for esketamine, a related compound administered as a nasal spray, when taken in combination with an oral antidepressant in patients who have not responded to other treatments. This seems to be a key point about the use of either ketamine or esketamine: it appears that they need to be part of an overall treatment program, which might include other medicines or non-medical approaches such as cognitive-behavioral therapy. The remarkable thing about the advent of esketamine, though, is that it was the first time a medicine with a new mechanism for treating depression was approved in perhaps thirty years.

Non-medical use of ketamine: A variety of animal studies have demonstrated ketamine's potential for dependence, and

---

[xv] It consequently increases the amount of glutamate that is available in the synapse (the space between neurons at their connecting points), and hence may alter the activity of other non-NMDA kinds of glutamate receptors, including the AMPA receptor. It also stimulates a type of opiate receptor (the 'mu' receptor), which likely contributes to its pain-reducing properties. Other effects involve receptors for other neurotransmitters, including those for monoamines and acetylcholine. Since pain relief often outlasts the duration which the drug is in the body, it seems likely that it produces an alteration of nerve cell function which continues for some time. It is not yet understood which combination of these qualities produces its clinical effects. One result of these actions, though, appears to be the formation of new connections between neurons ('synaptogenesis'), as we described earlier.

human research subjects describe its euphoric effects. It has been abused since the late 1970s, and in more recent years has been found in clubs, raves, and other settings, where it is sometimes called 'Vitamin K' or 'Special K.' Part of its popularity as a recreational drug comes from its rapidity of action, as well as the varied ways in which it can be taken, including by inhalation, oral ingestion, or injection. (Powders for inhalation or making into pills are derived from evaporating the injectable solution.) It often results in disorientation and hallucinations, which may be either pleasant or frightening. Deficits in coordination lead to a person moving very slowly and deliberately, and there is an increased likelihood of injury due to loss of pain sensation. It has been used as a date rape drug.

Tolerance develops to the dissociative and euphoric qualities of ketamine, and abrupt cessation from higher doses can result in a withdrawal syndrome including anxiety, excitation, very rapid heart rate, hallucinations, and shaking. It is classified as a Schedule III controlled substance by the Drug Enforcement Administration.

Etomidate: An antifungal medicine that made people sleepy

Etomidate was originally proposed as an antifungal drug, but because sedation was noticed in animal studies in the Janssen Pharmaceutica laboratories in 1964, it was later developed into an intravenous anesthetic which was approved in Europe in 1972 and the U.S. in 1983. It is given intravenously for induction of anesthesia, as well as for maintenance while using less potent agents such as nitrous oxide for brief surgical procedures.[xvi] In practice, it is often used for patients known to have fragile cardiovascular status. In the past, it was often given in emergency settings, though its use for this purpose declined after propofol became available. It generally has relatively limited effects on blood pressure and respiration but lacks analgesic properties. It also blocks synthesis of steroids in the adrenal gland, which can be of clinical concern, usually during longer periods of administration

Propofol: A new use for a chemical solvent

Propofol in the operating room: Propofol was developed by John B. Glen, a veterinary anesthesiologist and pharmacologist who was raised on a farm in western Scotland and trained at the University of Glasgow. Propofol had its roots as a solvent, as had trichloroethylene some decades earlier. Glen began developing it in 1973 at Imperial Chemical Industries, while looking at the effects of modifying the structures in a series of compounds known as *ortho*-alkylated phenols. His challenge when proposing it as an anesthetic was to convince his superiors that it sufficiently differed from the then-dominant thiopental in that it could not only induce anesthesia, but by careful continuous infusion could maintain it. It is very lipid-soluble, and cannot be dissolved in water but originally

---

[xvi] Etomidate acts by binding at sites on the $GABA_A$ receptor and potentiating the actions of GABA; hence, in a general sense it is similar in action to barbiturates.

was solubilized in a castor oil preparation. Clinical trials began in 1978 but were halted in 1980 after a number of deaths due to allergic reactions ('anaphylaxis'). Although the management was skeptical that there was any future for the drug, Glen argued forcefully that the deaths were related to the castor oil, not the drug itself. By 1984, he had developed a new formulation, involving an emulsion in soya oil. (Its milky color later led to it later being jokingly referred to as 'milk of amnesia.') This time clinical testing was very positive, and propofol was approved in Europe in 1986 and the U.S. in 1989.

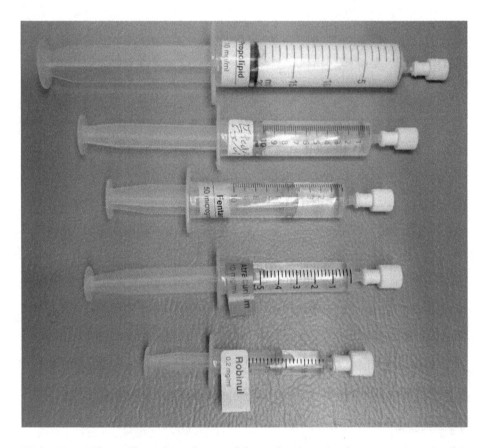

Figure 4-2: The milky color of propofol can be seen in the top syringe in this demonstration of typical medicines used during surgery in combination of the

volatile anesthetic sevoflurane (Chapter Five). Medicines seen here (top to bottom) are propofol for induction, ephedrine (in case of excessively low blood pressure), fentanyl (for pain), atracurium for neuromuscular blocking, and glycopyrronium bromide (Robinul) to reduce secretions.

Interestingly, ephedrine is a plant alkaloid from the Ephedra genus, another example of how plant alkaloids, known in general since ancient times (Chapter One), still find their way into modern life, often now in synthetic form.

The next challenge Glen faced was in finding a reliable way of maintaining infusions to make additional use of inhaled anesthetics less needed. He began work on a computer-driven apparatus, which later came to be known as Target-Controlled Infusion, in which desired blood levels, determined from mathematical modeling, are maintained. Once again, his superiors were hesitant to support it, and Glen instead put together international meetings at which colleagues could bring their expertise to its development. Finally, in 1993, his company gave it the go-ahead, and it is now used in many parts of the world, though not available in the U.S.

After its approval, propofol was rapidly accepted in view of its many desirable qualities. Among these was its rapid onset of action, often within thirty to forty-five seconds, and rapid awakening with minimal nausea when discontinued. Because it was administered intravenously, it transformed head and neck surgery, as the airway was not occupied as it would be with inhalational anesthetics. Its ease of use in carefully monitored outpatient settings also led to expansion of ambulatory surgery as well as procedures such as colonoscopy. It is used in general anesthesia induction, as well as sometimes for maintenance. It is also used for sedation, induction, and maintenance in patients on ventilators in intensive care settings, and in imaging studies requiring long periods of immobility. Currently it is found in the vast majority of surgical anesthesia inductions, and as of 2016, 190 million people are thought to have received it. Its mechanism of action continues to be studied.[xvii]

[xvii] Because propofol differs greatly from the drugs we have discussed previously, it's worthwhile to consider for a moment what is known about how it induces anesthesia. It seems likely that several mechanisms are involved. It at least partly involves stimulating a type of receptor for gamma aminobutyric acid (GABA), an inhibitory amino acid which plays a role in the sleep-inducing effects of barbiturates, benzodiazepines, and ethanol. It also blocks a type of channel which involves transport of sodium ions between the interior and outside of nerve cells, and it may also affect the system which responds to the active compounds in cannabis such as THC, as well as naturally occurring substances in the body which bind to the same receptors (Chapter Two). This 'endocannabinoid system' plays a role in sleep, memory, emotion, and reproduction. The relative degree to which these various possible mechanisms may affect propofol's properties as an anesthetic is not yet clearly understood.

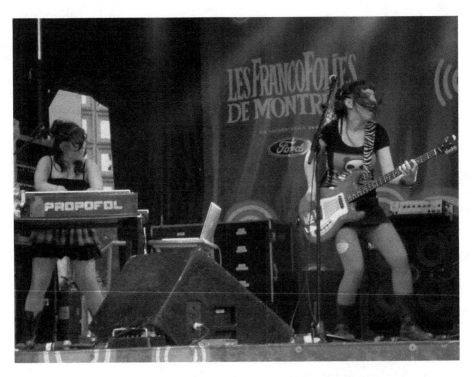

Figure 4-3: *Propofol is so ubiquitous, used in some 90 countries, that it has become something of a cultural icon. Here the musical group Propofol is performing in June 2012 in Montreal.*

Careful monitoring is of course important for safety reasons, as higher doses can suppress respiration and lower blood pressure, as well as affect cardiac function. Like thiopental, it induces sedation and unconsciousness but has little effect in reducing pain. Seizures may occur, and with longer-term use there is the rare possibility of propofol infusion syndrome, which involves metabolic changes, as well as cardiac and kidney failure. One well-known case of a fatality during propofol anesthesia was that of comedienne Joan Rivers, who experienced laryngospasm and cardiac arrest in 2014, when she was undergoing endoscopy and laryngoscopy to evaluate her hoarse voice and sore throat in an outpatient facility.

Propofol misuse and abuse: Propofol has potential for abuse, though it is uncommon, possibly because it can be hazardous with self-administration. Persons who have taken it in this manner have described pleasurable experiences, hallucinations, and sometimes heightening of sexual feelings. With repeated use, tolerance is thought to develop, so that increasing doses are needed to achieve the same effect. Addictive behavior is very uncommon, and, when it does occur, is frequently in anesthesiologists or other medical staff, possibly in those whose schedules include minimal periods of rest. It is not a Drug Enforcement Administration scheduled drug at this time.

Though propofol is clearly a euphoriant, some clinicians have the impression that it tends to be abused by persons with histories of sexual or other trauma, with a motivation of decreasing painful memories. Perhaps the most famous case of propofol misuse was that of Michael Jackson, who in the 1990s traveled accompanied by an anesthesiologist, and whose 2009 death was attributed to propofol given in combination with benzodiazepines ('Valium-like' sedatives). His doctor, who was later found guilty of involuntary manslaughter, reportedly said that Jackson's final words, apparently referring to propofol, were, 'Please give me my milk. I need my milk to sleep. It is the only thing that works.'[59]

Propofol and the relation of anesthesia to sleep: In the introduction, we talked about the relationship of anesthesia to sleep, commenting among other things that they differ in that in sleep, unlike anesthesia, a person usually can be aroused by stimuli (for instance, being touched or hearing one's name called), and has brain waves with complex cyclic patterns of REM and NREM sleep. Another important aspect of sleep is that, in addition to being influenced by the body clock, it is also affected by a homeostatic mechanism. This means that the body acts as if a certain amount of sleep is desirable, and that if a person gets less than that amount, he or she develops a 'sleep debt.' Later, if there is an opportunity, a person will sleep more to make up that debt. (For a fuller explanation, please see *The Science of Sleep*[60].)

Dr. Avery Tung and the author conducted studies at the University of Chicago to clarify the relationship of propofol anesthesia and sleep. It was found that when rats are sedated with propofol throughout their normal sleep time, and afterwards their brainwaves are studied, they do not have patterns suggesting that they were sleep deprived. This seemed to say that either propofol was keeping a sleep debt from accumulating or, alternatively, that during the anesthesia a sleep debt does not develop[61]. In another study, rats were sleep deprived, then half were placed under propofol anesthesia while the others were allowed to sleep. It was found that both groups recovered from the deprivation at the same rate.[62] One implication of this might be that after sleep deprivation in rats, recovery processes which occur during subsequent sleep can also occur while under anesthesia. There are, then, some similarities of sleep and anesthesia regarding how sleep is regulated homeostatically, but as we have described in the Introduction, there are also many differences between the two processes.

CHAPTER FIVE: POSTSCRIPT— MODERN HALOGENATED INHALATIONAL ANESTHETICS, THE 'Z' DRUGS, AND 21ST CENTURY MEDICINES FOR SLEEP

Halogenated inhalational anesthetics after halothane

The subsequent development of later agents is beyond the scope of this book, which focuses on the history of anesthetics found by individuals, often by happenstance, before the era in which these drugs became products of rational drug design conducted in a team setting. In order to give a sense of perspective, though, the following short comments describe the newer inhalational anesthetics, and more detail can be found in recent reviews[63].

Additional inhalational agents such as methoxyflurane and enflurane became available in the 1960s and early 1970s and played a role for the next two decades; methoxyflurane is no longer available in the U.S. and enflurane is rarely used. The modern agents most commonly employed now in the U.S. are isoflurane (1979), desflurane (1992), and sevoflurane (1992). As mentioned before, these were the results of manipulating molecules with specific goals in mind based on a knowledge of pharmacology. For example, Ross

C. Terrell (1925-2010) at Ohio Medical Products (part of Airco, Inc.), one of the developers of isoflurane, desflurane, and sevoflurane, guided his team to improve on halothane by using what are known as ether linkages. The rationale was that they were thought to have less likelihood of producing abnormal heart rhythms than the kind of structures contained in halothane[64]. In his early work, he also emphasized designing compounds with methyl-ethyl ether structures in particular, as they were thought to be more likely to have more selectively anesthetic properties.

Like halothane, these new compounds are volatile agents; that is, they are in liquid form at room temperature, and a vaporizer is used for making them suitable for inhalation. In general, their advantages are lower solubility (which improves both induction and recovery), potency, and minimal liver toxicity. They produce immobility and amnesia, but unlike nitrous oxide, they do not have analgesic properties. The choice among them is made by consideration of their various qualities including speed of induction, potency, clearance (rate of removal by the body), degree of metabolism to substances that might harm the liver, and side effect profile. Sevoflurane, for instance, is probably the most widely used agent in the U.S., partly due to having a sweet smell and relatively less airway irritation, while desflurane is less commonly used for induction due to its acrid odor and irritation, and it should not be administered for induction in children, whose more sensitive airways may develop spasm of the larynx.

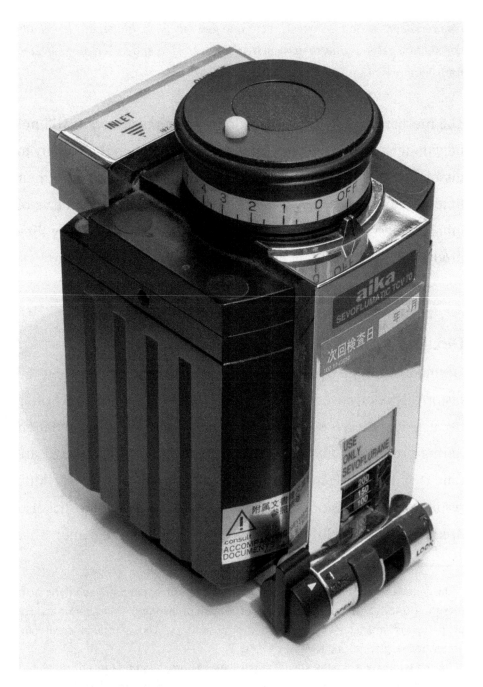

Figure 5-1: *Example of vaporizer apparatus. Isoflurane, desflurane, and sevoflurane are volatile anesthetics; that is, they are liquids at room temperature but can evaporate in order to be used as inhalational drugs. A vaporizer, as*

pictured here, is used to convert them into gaseous form. In contrast to volatile anesthetics, gaseous anesthetics such as nitrous oxide and xenon are delivered from compressed gas cylinders.

The mechanism by which inhalational anesthetics work is still not fully understood. In the past, interest has focused on their ability to dissolve in the lipid (fatty) membranes of neurons and alter their function. In the last few decades, interest turned to the effects of inhaled anesthetics on drug receptors.[xviii,65]. The precise way they produce their effects remains to be established.

Dexmedetomidine

Dexmedetomidine was developed in 1999, and hence is beyond the historical period covered in this book, but is being mentioned briefly because it represented a new mechanism for producing sedation during procedures and in intubated patients in the intensive care unit. [xix] It has analgesic properties and produces relatively little respiratory suppression, though it can lower blood pressure. It is also used off-label for delirium, alcohol withdrawal, and in conjunction

---

[xviii] In general, they augment the activity of a type of gamma aminobutyric acid receptor ('GABA$_A$'), as well as some types of potassium channels, while altering activity of pathways mediated by other neurotransmitters. These include serotonin, acetylcholine, glycine, and NMDA.

[xix] Dexmedetomidine acts by stimulating a type of norepinephrine receptor ('alpha-2'), which decreases sympathetic nervous system activity. This largely involves neurons involving norepinephrine in the brainstem (the 'locus coeruleus') and spinal cord. Thus, it is very different than benzodiazepines and barbiturates, whose action is primarily on GABA$_A$ receptors, particularly in the hypothalamus.

with analgesics. It is unlike most induction agents, in that its effects are typically not evident for five to ten minutes

Dexmedetomidine is not recommended for use longer than twenty-four hours, though it is sometimes given in this manner. When it is given for longer periods, discontinuation can sometimes produce agitation, or nausea and vomiting.

Dexmedetomidine is also interesting in that it has been reported to produce EEG patterns similar to N2 ('stage 2') NREM sleep in children having nuclear medicine studies.[66] It is sometimes used off-label to increase sleep at night in non-intubated adults in the ICU setting [67], with a goal of reducing the likelihood of developing delirium, a common occurrence which may partially be due to sleep deprivation. The recordings, however, showed no increase in N3 ('slow-wave sleep') compared to placebo and essentially no REM sleep. Moreover, there was no clear decrease in the rate of development of delirium. Although the length of stay in the ICU was lower, the overall stay in the hospital was longer. Some authors have pointed out that in the absence of more typical sleep architecture, or any noticeable gain in the restorative qualities associated with sleep, it is unclear whether the state induced by dexmedetomidine should be considered sleep or sedation.[68] Perhaps the most significant point about dexmedetomidine for the purposes of this book is that it is a reminder that there are many different neurophysiological routes by which drugs produce sedation and anesthesia.

Medicines for sleep since the 1980s

The 'Z drugs': Sleep medicines, like those for anesthesia, continued to grow apart in the 1980s. In efforts to maximize the benefits and reduce the liabilities of benzodiazepines, companies used new knowledge of the structure of the $GABA_A$ receptor to design compounds whose effects were more specific to sleep. While benzodiazepines were found to bind to a wide range of types of receptor subunits ('alpha 1,2,3 and 5'), newer drugs were developed which tended to focus on the alpha 1 subunit, which in animal studies was thought to be most specific for sleep. Among these were zaleplon, zolpidem, and zopiclone, which became available in the 1980s and early 1990s, and eszopiclone (the active portion of zopiclone) appeared in the U.S. in 2004. They were perceived to be advantageous in terms of having a higher degree of action on sleep compared to effects on memory, coordination, and muscle relaxation.

Individual comparisons of efficacy varied as to whether the new drugs were indeed more effective for sleep, and some suggested that they were about the same. To use the example of zopiclone, for instance, a large analysis of multiple studies found their benefits comparable[69]. A report of the U.K. National Institute for Health Care and Excellence reported that, although definitive data were lacking, 'currently there was no compelling evidence of a clinically useful difference between the Z drugs and shorter-acting benzodiazepine hypnotics from the point of view of their effectiveness, adverse effects, or potential for dependence or abuse'.[70] Similarly, a 2008 survey of patients in the UK found that they experienced no difference in terms of the benefits or side effects of benzodiazepines and Z drugs, although patients taking the latter more often desired to stop the medicine.[71] Others have noted the apparently lower rate of tolerance and abuse potential in Z drugs compared to benzodiazepines. [72] The clinical impression from practical experience in a large study of European family practitioners and pharmacists indicated that they favored Z drugs in terms of both efficacy and safety, perhaps, the author commented, more so than is borne out of rigorous laboratory studies[73].

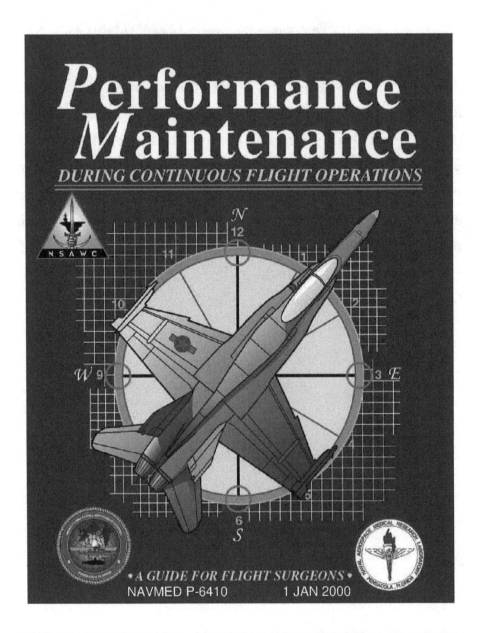

Figure 5-2: U.S. Navy guide for flight surgeons regarding sleep and sleep medicines. The military and the transportation industry have an ongoing concern about the effects of inadequate sleep, as well as the potential benefits and risks of hypnotics, on performance. As of 2012, the U.S. Air Force guidelines listed two Z drugs and one benzodiazepine as 'no-go' pills; that is, medicines which can be

taken in the sleep period before flying, each with a certain minimum number of hours required before flight.[74]

21st century medicines for sleep: Since the 2000s, at least three new hypnotics have appeared which are intriguing because they differ from the benzodiazepines and Z drugs in that they do not produce their actions by alterations of GABA$_A$ receptor function. Ramelteon (Rozerem, 2005), which acts as an agonist at melatonin receptors, primarily has effects on the time it takes to fall asleep. Doxepin for sleep (Silenor, 2010) represents a new application of low doses of an antidepressant which has been available since the 1960s and is primarily oriented to improving awakenings during the night. Suvorexant (Belsomra, 2014), which acts by inhibiting the action of the neurotransmitters known as orexins, is used both for difficulties initiating and maintaining sleep. At the time of this writing, other 'dual orexin receptor antagonist' hypnotics are in development. As mentioned earlier, both the Z drugs and these newer compounds are outside the period covered in this history and are mentioned here for the sake of completeness and context. Detailed descriptions of their mechanisms, benefits, and limitations can be found in the companion book *Understanding Sleeping Pills.*[75]

CHAPTER SIX: SUMMARY

So far, we have covered a great deal of human history and the development of many different drugs along the way to modern agents for sleep and anesthesia. In conclusion, let's look again at the similarities and differences between the two and the medicines which produce them. Then, in order to make it easier to see each step in the history of medicines in relation to each other, and help give a sense of context, it might be useful to summarize this whole history in just a few pages. Then we'll go on to thoughts about the movement from plant-based to synthetic drugs, some of the qualities of the people who made the discoveries, the element of chance in their findings, and the movement from discoveries by individuals to the fruits of team efforts using rational drug design.

Sleep and anesthesia

Sleep and general anesthesia have one overriding similarity, in that they both involve unconsciousness and reduced responsiveness to the outside world. They are both reversible in the sense that the sleeper spontaneously awakens, as does the anesthetized patient when the medicine is stopped. In this sense, this distinguishes them from coma, which may involve unconsciousness and loss of responsiveness for weeks or months or longer. Sleep and anesthesia also have differences. The EEG of sleep shows a highly regulated pattern of approximately ninety-minute cyclic changes between NREM and REM sleep, whereas anesthesia manifests a relatively consistent pattern of slowing without cyclic processes and varying degrees of slow waves depending on depth. A sleeper can be aroused by sensory stimuli, whereas a patient under anesthetic cannot. During sleep, there may be some fluctuations in blood pressure and respiration (especially during REM), but in general anesthesia they may be profoundly depressed.

Just as the two states have both similarities and differences, so do the medicines which produce them. Some medicines such as barbiturates and benzodiazepines have been taken orally for sleep, but when given intravenously they have been used for anesthesia induction or sedation. The distinction between the two types of medicines became clearer in the 1960s and subsequently with the development of intravenous anesthetics beginning with the dissociative agent ketamine and continuing with etomidate and propofol. Animal studies with propofol, however, have suggested that the boundaries of sleep and anesthesia need further exploration. It turns out, for instance, that recovery from prior sleep deprivation can occur during prolonged propofol anesthesia (see Chapter Four).

The effects of drugs on sedation/sleep are often misunderstood. Through much of history, opiates were considered sleep promoters;

in modern times, it has been found that the state of seeming somnolence after acute administration is often more like profound sedation than sleep, and indeed opiates may actually prolong the time it takes to fall asleep or increase awakenings during the night (see Chapter Two). This kind of misunderstanding sometimes appears to this day. There have been claims, for instance, that dexmedetomidine produces stage 2 sleep, while others have pointed out that the EEG lacks any increase in slow-wave sleep or virtually any REM sleep, have noted the absence of any sleep-like restoration, and have questioned whether the state most closely resembles sleep or sedation. The misuse of anesthetics to produce sleep can also lead to tragic consequences, as in the extreme case of Michael Jackson's reliance on propofol and subsequent death. Another kind of distinction between medicines for sleep and anesthesia is that although typically a single medicine is given for sleep, general anesthesia, at least in longer and more complicated surgeries, usually requires the combined use of several drugs, including ones for induction and maintenance, as well as muscle relaxants and pain medicines.

Brief summary of the history of drugs for sleep and anesthesia

Psychoactive substances first appeared in pre-history, as plants evolved alkaloids, substances which, along with other possible functions, served as mechanisms of defense against predators. They were, in effect, 'chemical thorns' which might incapacitate an animal or person by intoxication, sedation, or toxicity. Many of these became recognized as hallucinogens or intoxicants; others evolved into medicines for sleep or pain.

In early civilizations, illness was often seen in religious terms, for instance, as punishment for sin. Not surprisingly, medicines began to be seen in the same light and were often involved in sacrificial ceremonies in which collective guilt was transferred to some unlucky animal, or alternatively to humans, who were then exiled or worse. In time, this process became more and more symbolic, but the association of medicines with religion persisted. The early Greek word for medicines, for instance, is related to the word for scapegoat; even our modern words such as 'pharmacy' and 'pharmacist' evolved from roots involving magic and sorcery.

By the time of classical Greece, hallucinogens and sedatives were tied up in both healing and religion. The sick flocked to the temples of Asclepius, where drug-induced intoxication and sleep would lead to dreams which were interpreted by the priests to suggest the path to health. Seers at the temple of Apollo would become intoxicated by alkaloids or naturally formed gases such as ethylene (later an anesthetic in the early 20th century), and then give highly valued pronouncements about the future. In the cult of Dionysus, hallucinogens produced by ergot fungi were involved in the ecstatic religious ceremonies.

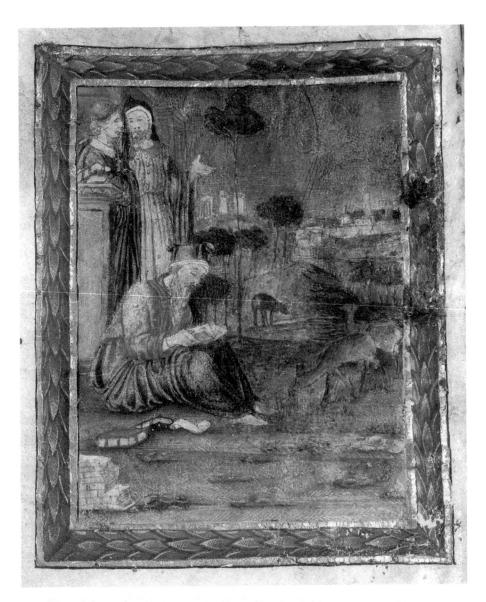

Figure 6-1: In this depiction, Hippocrates (c460-c370 BC) is reading while seated, and behind him two philosophers seem to have strong feelings about their conversation. This is from an illustration in a 15ᵗʰ century manuscript of Hippocrates' Aphorisms. His collected sayings have survived and continue to be read. Examples: 'Both sleep and insomnolency, when immoderate, are bad.' 'Life is short and Art long; the crisis fleeting; experience perilous, and decisions difficult.' (Hippocrates: Aphorisms. The Perfect Library, publishers, 2015)

It was into this atmosphere that the physician Hippocrates of Kos had a revolutionary idea—sickness was not necessarily a punishment from on high, but rather a disorder of the body's processes. It followed, then, that drugs did not produce their effects by mystical means, but rather by making alterations in the body which could be studied and understood. He also recognized that there was decreased pain sensation during unconsciousness and used the word anesthesia, though its meaning was more related to lack of sensation due to disease. He believed that opium was not magical, but that by altering physiological processes it produced sedation and reduction in pain.

Through the post-classical period and into the Middle Ages, drugs— often opiates and plant alkaloids—were dispensed by persons considered to be witches and sorcerers, until the rise of universities in the 11th and 12th centuries which added new societal respectability to studying drugs. Surgery was often performed while having a patient breathe through a *spongia somnifera*, a cloth impregnated with opium, mandrake, henbane, and hemlock.

In the 1500s, the Swiss physician Paracelsus heralded a new way of medical thinking, signaling his desire to look forward instead of to the past. To this end, he lectured in German instead of Latin and put up announcements of his lectures with invitations to all—not just academics—in a way that reminded some of Martin Luther's posting of his theses on the church door in Wittenberg. He believed that individual medicines should be developed for specific illnesses rather than looking for grand panaceas. He also reported the analgesic properties of ether in animal experiments, though this did not progress to humans until the 19th century. These new approaches and ways of thinking were all part of a larger movement which came to be known as the Medical Renaissance and laid the foundations for modern medicine.

By the early 19th century, the main agents available to aid sleep or provide anesthesia were still compounds with ancient roots. The effects of cannabis on sleep in the short term are unclear, and chronic use leads to sleep disturbance. Though the use of cannabis in surgery had roots in ancient India and China, it never gained wide acceptance for this purpose in the West, where it and its modern derivatives continue to receive growing interest for other medical applications. Alkaloids such as mandrake and henbane were relatively ineffective, and very toxic. Surgeons were limited primarily to two agents—ethyl alcohol and opium.

Alcohol is no friend of sleep. Any benefit from shortening the time to fall asleep is outweighed by disrupted sleep later at night as blood levels fall. And similar to cannabis, its chronic use leads to long-term sleep disturbance. In terms of oral use by itself for surgery, alcohol, like substances such as mandrake and henbane, reflects an ancient motivation to use intoxication as a remedy for surgical pain. But intoxication itself is generally of limited effectiveness and was a poor substitute for anesthesia.

Opium clearly produces a somnolent-appearing state of sedation, but it actually disturbs nighttime sleep with increasing arousals and sometimes taking even longer to fall asleep. As with alcohol, dependent persons complain of difficulty sleeping, unrefreshing sleep, and daytime sleepiness. Both alcohol and opiates are poor choices for surgical anesthesia when given by themselves, as the doses needed for true anesthesia, with qualities such as immobility, lack of response to stimuli, and lack of pain sensation, are not achieved until the toxic range, which can easily become lethal due to respiratory arrest or other causes. As we will see later, in modern anesthesia, the analgesic benefits of opiates are achieved by giving lower doses in combination with other drugs for induction, muscle relaxation, and maintenance of anesthesia.

It was in this setting that both new inhalational anesthetics as well as synthetic agents for sleep began to make their appearance in the mid-19th century and beyond. Nitrous oxide, with roots in the late 18th century, and ether, going back to the medical renaissance and rediscovery by Faraday in 1818, were first used primarily for recreation, and their medical application did not appear until the 1840s.

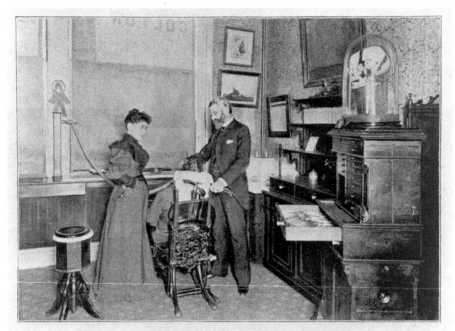

DR. NEVIUS IN THE ACT OF ADMINISTERING NITROUS OXIDE GAS, COLTON DENTAL
ASSOCIATION, COOPER INSTITUTE, NEW YORK.

Figure 6-2: *Nitrous oxide being given to a dental patient, 1894,*

Nitrous oxide was limited in its potency, and though ether was revolutionary as a surgical anesthetic, its shortcomings included its unpleasant odor, volatility which could fill the room and affect staff, irritation to the airway, and explosiveness. Chloroform, which had been discovered in 1831 by several people, including Samuel Guthrie, who was looking to make a pesticide by distilling chlorinated lime with whiskey, began to see clinical use in obstetric anesthesia in the late 1840s. It had a more rapid onset and more pleasant odor, was easier to administer, and was less flammable, but it required more skill to avoid toxicity. A great deal of experience was gained with chloroform during the American Civil War and then the

Boer War, and it was widely used until the advent of intravenous barbiturates and marginally safer inhaled anesthetics in the early part of the 20th century.

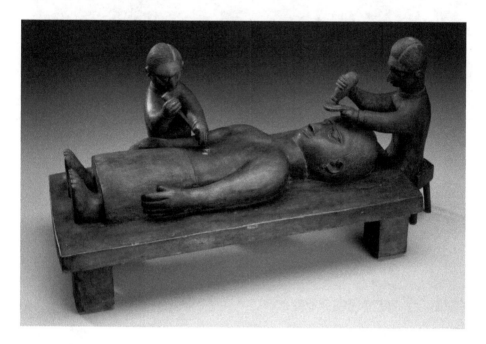

Figure 6-3: Abdominal surgery using ether or chloroform dripped onto a mask over the patient's mouth and nose. The wooden carving was given to a Dr. Simpson, a medical officer in Cameroon, portraying him performing the surgery, in 1925.

The success of chloroform led to the search for a more palatable oral agent and culminated in the clinical utilization of chloral hydrate in 1869. It was a milestone in the sense that it was the first sedative which was not plant-derived but rather wholly synthetic. Though the theory behind its functionality was incorrect—it was mistakenly thought to be metabolized to chloroform—it was one of the first steps in a tradition of what came to be known as synthetic organic chemistry, with roots in the synthesis of urea in 1828 and the synthetic dye industry in the 1850s. Barbituric acid was created in 1864, though a clinically used barbiturate did not appear until 1903.

In the early part of the 20th century, several new inhalational anesthetics became available. In 1908, it was noticed that when gas fixtures were used for lighting in the botanical gardens at the University of Chicago, the carnation flowers wilted. The culprit turned out to be one of its constituents, ethylene, which, when coming from natural sources, may have intoxicated the seers at the Temple of Apollo in ancient Greece (Prologue), and which had been synthesized in the 18th century. Arno Luckhardt and J. Bailey Carter at the University of Chicago studied it and noted its soporific qualities in animals. After assuring themselves of its safety by inhaling it themselves multiple times, they turned it over for clinical use to the Presbyterian Hospital in Chicago, and they later made it available to the medical profession without patent or monetary gain.

Ethylene was followed by cyclopropane in the late 1920s and 1930s, but its use was limited by its flammability and the tendency to cause abnormal heart rhythms and disastrous drops in blood pressure known as 'cyclopropane shock.' Trichloroethylene, synthesized in the 19th century and used as a metal degreaser, was developed as an anesthetic in the late 1930s and 1940s. Though having the advantage of being less flammable, it turned out that it was metabolized into toxic substances which caused nerve palsies. Its use declined after the development of halothane in the 1950s and isoflurane in the late 1970s.

The second half of the 20th century saw the development of three remarkable intravenous anesthetics. The benzodiazepine ('Valium-like') drugs were discovered in the late 1950s by Leo Sternbach, a chemist at the Hoffman LaRoche laboratories in New Jersey, who had been using fabric dyes from his training days as the building blocks for possible new tranquilizers. He was told by his boss to move on to other projects, but a few years later, when an assistant came across one of the old bottles while cleaning the laboratory, Sternbach decided to run it through behavioral tests. It proved to have tranquilizing effects in animals and later humans, and it was ultimately marketed as Librium in 1960. It and later benzodiazepines rapidly became widely used as tranquilizers, anticonvulsants, and sleeping pills. Intravenous midazolam found a place in anesthesia, for perioperative sedation and induction, as well as sedation during diagnostic procedures or for intubated patients in the intensive care unit. Limitations of oral benzodiazepines became apparent as the years went on. Their oral use for sleep declined with the advent of the 'Z drugs' such as zolpidem in the late 1980s and 1990s, and their function as tranquilizers continues to decline in favor of SSRI antidepressants. The use of midazolam for anesthesia induction greatly declined with the later development of propofol, but it is widely used for sedation during uncomfortable procedures and related purposes.

Ketamine, approved in the U.S. in 1970, is used as an induction agent followed by other anesthetics, or as the sole anesthetic if muscle relaxation is not required, and for outpatient procedures in which patients are not intubated. Its advantages include the rapidity of onset and minimal reductions of blood pressure. Unlike earlier agents, it can cause hallucinations and dissociation reactions in which patients describe out-of-body experiences. These are often minimized by concomitant use of benzodiazepines. In more recent years, it has come to be used off-label in psychiatry for rapid improvement in patients who have not responded to other antidepressants, and the related compound esketamine, applied intranasally, was approved for this use in 2019.

Propofol, derived from a solvent, was developed in the late 1970s by John B. Glen, a veterinary anesthesiologist and pharmacologist at Imperial Chemical Industries, who first had to convince his bosses that it was fundamentally distinct in its properties from thiopental. After deaths due to allergic reactions to the castor oil in which it was originally suspended, the company at first planned to discontinue it, but he rescued the drug by developing a new preparation with soy oil. Propofol was rapidly accepted, in part because of its rapid onset and offset, with less emergence difficulties such as nausea and vomiting. Since it was intravenous, it made it much easier do some forms of head and neck surgery without the use of inhalational anesthetics. It found a place as an induction agent, for maintenance in shorter operations, and as a form of sedation for patients on ventilators. It continues to be the most common agent used in surgical induction

The second half of the 20th century also saw the advent of improved inhalational anesthetics, in a sense derivatives of ether, which grew later into the agents still used today. The first of these came from the work of Charles Walter Suckling, in an effort to find agents which improved on both ether and chloroform, as well as the relatively newer cyclopropane and trichloroethylene. Benefitting from knowledge of halogen chemistry gleaned from atomic bomb research and realizing that adding halogen atoms such as fluorine or chlorine increased potency and reduced flammability, he came up with halothane in 1951. Its benefits included not being irritating to the airway and not being explosive. It could, however, produce abnormal heart rhythms and respiratory depression, as well as liver damage, which came to be known as 'halothane hepatitis.' From the late 1970s onward, it fell into disuse in favor of newer agents. It is no longer available in the U.S. but holds an important place as a precursor to these newer inhaled anesthetics. It is also important in that it was one of the first cases in anesthesia of what came to be known as rational drug design; that is, purposefully synthesizing drugs on the basis of what has been learned about the pharmacologic effects of changing their structure, as well as knowledge of physiology or disease processes.

From the late 1970s through the 1990s, newer halogenated inhalational anesthetics were developed, including isoflurane, desflurane, and sevoflurane. They improved on halothane in terms of potency, lower rates of liver toxicity, and lower solubility into tissues, which improves speed of onset and offset. They remain the main inhalational anesthetics today, particularly sevoflurane. Preferences for a particular agent among them is often based on potency, rate of removal from the body, side effect profile, and other factors. As we described earlier, they are usually given as part of a combination of drugs, beginning with an induction agent such as propofol, a muscle relaxant, the inhalational anesthetic for maintenance, and pain medication.

The movement from plant-based to synthetic drugs

As we described in Chapter One, from prehistory on, substances that became medicines (for instance, quinine, quinidine, opiates) were derived from plant alkaloids. Other alkaloids remain part of modern life (caffeine, nicotine) or continue as drugs of abuse (cocaine, again opiates). Alkaloids remained the dominant source of medicines until well into the 19th century. As detailed in a companion book, *Molecules, Madness, and Malaria*[76], the discovery of synthetic fabric dyes in 1856 led to the development of an industry which took advantage of its newfound skills in synthetic organic chemistry to branch out into a variety of directions, including the development of paints, food colorings, agricultural chemicals, and medicines. Among the first synthetic drugs which appeared in the 19th century were methylene blue (first developed as a fabric dye) and chloral hydrate, the first fully synthetic sedative. As we saw in Chapter Four, the legacy of fabric dyes evolving into sedatives persisted into modern times, when Leo Sternbach used previously unsuccessful dyes as the building blocks for what became the benzodiazepine tranquilizers, sleeping pills, and anesthetics.

Samuel Guthrie hadn't realized the composition of the chloroform he synthesized, and initially the clinical discoverers of chloral hydrate were mistaken about its route of breakdown, but over time as skills advanced there was better understanding of chemical structure and metabolism. By the late 20th century, syntheses become more complex and began to be driven by knowledge of how manipulation of molecules might have specific pharmacologic effects. There was a movement from discovery by individuals to the setting of teams of scientists working in large pharmaceutical companies. We will come back to this, but first let us look a bit at some of the remarkable people who found the earlier medicines for sleep and anesthesia.

The discoverers

In one sense, they were very different from each other. Samuel Guthrie, restless in his life as a rural physician, indulged his fascination with chemistry in a backyard laboratory, where he tinkered with improving methods of preparing gunpowder, molasses, and pesticides, and stumbled upon chloroform.

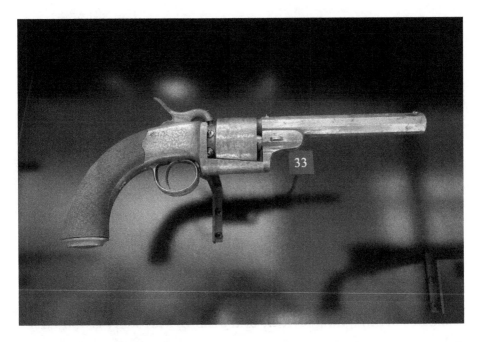

Figure 6-4: Percussion cap revolver, about 1850: Samuel Guthrie is known not only for chloroform, but also for developing 'S. Guthrie's Waterproof Percussion Priming', a step toward a new system of priming firearms. This led ultimately to the demise of flintlock guns, which were fired by a spark produced by flint striking steel. Guthrie's business in priming powder was successful, but led to multiple explosions in his facility, in one of which he was injured badly. The later development of percussion firearms has an intriguing history, with major advances made in 1840 by a Scottish clergyman, Alexander Forsyth, and in 1845 by Baltimore dentist Edward Maynard.

William Morton was a dentist with a shady past, whose motivation in introducing ether was to monetize it for his private gain. James Simpson, in contrast, seemed driven to find something to relieve suffering. He was a deeply religious man, and one can imagine his feeling when accused publicly of going against biblical teachings. As we described before, Arno Luckhardt and J. Bailey Carter, concerned about the safety of his idea of using ethylene, tested it on themselves 700 times before releasing it for general clinical use, and in contrast to William Morton, made it available for free and without patent to the medical community. Leo Sternbach, a chemist who had known antisemitism in Poland and fled Hitler's aggrandizement in Europe, had a genuine love for medicinal chemistry, was a bit too free in his willingness to show disdain for his superiors, and was motivated by a desire to be left alone to pursue his chemical interests wherever they might take him. John B. Glen grew up on a farm and went on to study veterinary medicine and, ultimately, pain relief. Even when winning the Lasker award in his old age, he was still prone to use analogies of ploughing furrows and dealing with stony ground. Like Simpson, his fellow Scot, he had an impulse to dig down and keep going in the face of criticism or adversity, as he put it, to 'persevere in hope.'[77]

Though these discoverers had different backgrounds and personalities, they also seemed to share some traits, notably the courage of their convictions and independence. In ancient Greece, when both illnesses and drugs were deeply embedded in religious and magical lore, it must have taken a great deal of self-assurance for Hippocrates to argue that drugs could be understood without benefit of magic but rather in terms of their effects on body physiology. Two millennia later, when scholarship was understood to involve reading and re-reading the wisdom of the ancients, Paracelsus took the brave and symbolic step of challenging them, even at one point burning their works, and turning instead to the what could be learned from new observations. In doing so, he also took the revolutionary stance that wisdom could be found outside clerical and academic sources in the collective experience of barber-surgeons and apothecaries. In a sense, this was even more challenging than for Hippocrates, who was accepted as an Asclepiad physician and teacher. Paracelsus, in contrast, was without such a home, and although he briefly lectured at the University of Basel, he spent most of his career as an itinerant physician, traveling from city to city to learn and to teach. In some senses, one of his descendants was Henri Laborit, who a half a millennium later revolutionized psychiatric practice in the 1950s with the clinical discovery of chlorpromazine (Thorazine) in a career outside of traditional academic institutions.[78]

As drug development became more and more performed inside large pharmaceutical corporations, some of the discoveries still carried the marks of individual tenacity. Leo Sternbach had been told by his superiors at Hoffman LaRoche to stop working on tranquilizers and instead to study antibiotics, when a few years later he came across an old bottle from his previous work and had it tested for behavioral effects. The result was the first of the benzodiazepines. One is reminded of Frank Berger at Wallace Laboratories, whose administration was skeptical that his proposal for meprobamate, a drug to reduce anxiety, would have a market. Undaunted, Berger made a movie of its effects on animals, presented it at a major medical meeting, and amidst the resulting enthusiasm got the go-ahead for producing meprobamate (Miltown), which became one of the first 'blockbuster' drugs in psychiatry.[79] In the late 1970s, John B.

Glen had a difficult time persuading his superiors at Imperial Chemical Industries that his new drug propofol was sufficiently unlike the widely used thiopental to make it worth developing. As we mentioned earlier, when later deaths occurred and the company was in favor of abandoning it, Glen successfully convinced them that the fatalities were due to allergic reactions to the particular oil in which it was immersed, not to the drug itself, and he found a new preparation which avoided this problem. He then, once again facing initial skepticism from his bosses, developed the computer-driven Target-Controlled Infusion system for its administration. Ultimately, propofol became the most widely administered drug for anesthesia induction in the world.

Serendipitous discoveries

Much has been made of the role of chance events in psychopharmacology (see companion book *The Curious History of Medicines in Psychiatry*), and serendipity appears here too. What if Samuel Guthrie had not inadvertently synthesized chloroform while trying to make a related compound and noticed its soporific effects? Simpson got the idea of using chloroform for anesthesia during a chance conversation in 1847 with physician/chemist David Waldie, who told him that when patients inhaled a particular asthma remedy, they tended to become sleepy, and its potential was mentioned. Though these were chance events, they happened to people who were prepared to see their implications and go where they led them. In the 1920s, Arno Luckhardt and J. Bailey Carter were exploring why burning illuminating gas in a greenhouse caused carnation flowers to close and came up with ethylene as an anesthetic. In the 1960s, researchers noticed that patients receiving an antifungal drug became sleepy, leading to the development of etomidate as an anesthetic. We mentioned Leo Sternbach's discovery of benzodiazepines earlier under the topic of tenacity, but chance also played a role: it was his assistant's finding of an old bottle of a fabric dye derivative that led to his testing the compound that became chlordiazepoxide.

Discoveries became more and more team efforts

As we have just summarized, the history of discoveries of drugs for sleep and anesthesia often involved the serendipitous observations of individuals. During the second half of the 20th century, this began to change. Partly this was due to the increasing complexity of syntheses; it was less likely by then that a new anesthetic could be made, as was chloroform in 1831, by distilling chlorinated lime and whiskey. More elaborate work required increasingly sophisticated laboratory equipment and teams of people with complementary skills, often in large pharmaceutical companies. As we just saw, even in this setting, some discoveries carried the mark of individuals, notably Leo Sternbach's discovery of benzodiazepines at Hoffman LaRoche in the 1950s, and John B. Glen's development of propofol at Imperial Chemical Industries in the 1970s. Another would be Charles Walter Suckling's work on halothane at Imperial Chemical Industries in the 1950s.

This trend to discovery by teams, though often led by very talented individuals, reflected not only increasing complexity of procedures, but also the growth of rational drug design. As mentioned earlier, Suckling, in developing halothane, was armed in advance with the knowledge that adding halogen atoms to hydrocarbon molecules designed for anesthesia would likely make them less flammable. Ross Terrell, in developing many of the newer halogenated anesthetics including isoflurane, desflurane, and sevoflurane, was able to guide his team to design compounds with ether linkages, which were thought to produce fewer cardiac arrhythmias. Once again, this approach often requires screening large numbers of compounds (desflurane which came to market in the early 1990s, for instance, was number 653), more suitable to the resources of large corporations, in that case, Airco, Inc. There is also a matter of expense. Currently companies maintain 'chemical libraries' of huge quantities of molecules, which can be assessed in high-throughput screening procedures performing literally millions of tests. The median cost of research and development of a new drug brought to market from 2009-2018 has been estimated to be $985 million.[80]

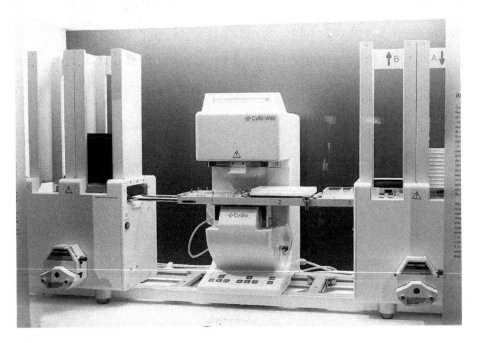

Figure 6-5: Example of a high-throughput screening device. Information gleaned from this technique, for instance determining that a specific part of a molecule may relate to a particular pharmacological action, can then be applied to drug design. High-throughput screening is also used in many other industries involving oil and gas, food and agriculture and materials testing.

The move to the work of teams comprised of members with overlapping skills and using the approach of rational drug design in the mid-to-late 20th century was seen in other areas of pharmacology as well. As mentioned earlier, in psychiatry the change was exemplified by the advent of the SSRI antidepressant fluoxetine (Prozac) at the Eli Lilly company in the 1980s, based on the monoamine hypothesis, which suggested that increasing amounts of brain substances such as serotonin might improve depression.[81] This shift has been very productive, and it continues to produce newer anesthetics and medicines in many different areas. At the same time, it's also good to remember an earlier era in which many of the landmark medicines were discovered, often with an element of chance, by some observant, persevering, and often colorful individuals.

ACKNOWLEDGEMENTS

I would like to thank Richard Roger CRNA, MEd, MS for his helpful comments and suggestions. Any errors which remain are my own.

PICTURE CREDITS

Cover illustration: (Stages in the production of ether showing various retorts in use on furnaces. Engraving 17__) From the Wellcome Collection, under Attribution 4.0 International (CC BY 4.0) license.

Fig. 1-1: (Ephedra): Prof. Otto Wilhelm Thomé: *Flora von Deutschland, Osterreich und der Schweitz*, 1885. From Wikimedia Commons, which states 'Permission granted to use under GFDL by Kurt Stueber.' 'This work is in the public domain in the United States because it was published (or registered with the U.S. Copyright office) before January 1, 1925.'

Fig. 1-2: (Temple at Delphi): Kris Silver, from Wikimedia Commons, in the public domain under Creative Commons Share-Alike 3.0 unported license.

Fig. 1-3: (Paracelsus): Copy of painting by Quentin Matsys, from Wikimedia Commons, in the public domain in the country of origin and other countries and areas where the copyright term is the author's life plus 70 years or fewer.

Fig. 2-1: (Hua Tuo) From the Wellcome Collection, in the public domain by Attribution 4.0 International (CC BY 4.0).

Fig. 2-2: (Samuel Colt): John Chester Buttre, from Wikimedia Commons, which states 'This media file is in the public domain in the United States. This applies to U.S. works where the copyright has expired, often because its first publication occurred prior to January 1, 1925, and if not then due to lack of notice or renewal.'

Fig. 2-3: (Humphry Davy): Humphry Davy's experience breathing nitrous oxide at the Pneumatic Institute of Clifton, by Louis Figuler, 1868. From Wikimedia Commons, which states 'This work is in the public domain in the United States because it was published (or registered with the U.S. Copyright office) before January 1, 1925.'

Fig. 2-4: (Morton's ether inhaler): From the Wellcome Collection under Creative Commons Attribution 4.0 (CC BY 4.0) terms and conditions.

Fig. 2-5: (Crawford Long postage stamp): U.S. Post Office. From Wikimedia Commons, which states 'This work is in the public domain in the United States because it is a work prepared by an officer or employee of the United States Government as part of that person's official duties under the term of Title 17, Chapter 1, Section 105 of the U.S. Code.'

Fig. 2-6: (John Snow's chloroform inhaler). From the Wellcome Collection under Creative Commons Attribution 4.0 (CC BY 4.0) terms and conditions.

Fig. 2-7: (Portable anesthetic kit): From the Science Museum, London and the Wellcome Collection, under Attribution 4.0 International (CC BY 4.0) license.

Fig. 3-1: (ethylene apparatus). From Luckhardt, A.B. and Carter, J.B.: Ethylene as a gas anesthetic. Current Res. Anesthesia & Analgesia 2: 221-229, 1923. This work is in the public domain in the United States because it was published (or registered with the U.S. Copyright office) before January 1, 1925.

Fig. 3-2: (gas centrifuge). Fastfission, from Wikimedia Commons, which states 'Fastfission grants anyone the right to use this work for any purpose, without any conditions, unless such conditions are required by law.'

Fig. 4-1: (University of Krakow): Iwona Grabska, from Wikimedia Commons, in the public domain under Creative Commons Share-Alike 3.0 Unported License.

Fig. 4-2: (Propofol syringe): Mikael Haggstrom, from Wikimedia Commons, in the public domain under Creative Commons CC 1.0 Universal Public Domain Dedication.

Fig. 4-3: (Propofol band). Jeangagnon, from Wikimedia Commons, in the public domain under Creative Commons Share-Alike 4.0 International License.

Fig. 5-1: (Vaporizer): Ignis, from Wikimedia Commons, in the public domain under the terms of the GNU free documentation license version 1.2 or any later version published by the Free Software Foundation.

Fig. 5-2: (Guide for flight surgeons): U.S. Navy, Bureau of Medicine and Surgery: Performance maintenance during continuous flight operations: a guide for flight surgeons, January 1, 2000. From Wikimedia Commons, which states 'This work is in the public domain in the United States because it is a work prepared by an officer or employee of the United States Government as part of that person's official duties under the term of Title 17, Chapter 1, Section 105 of the U.S. Code.'

Fig. 6-1: (Hippocrates) From Wikimedia Commons and Wellcome Images, under Creative Commons Attribution 4.0 International License.

Fig. 6-2: (nitrous oxide being given to a dental patient): Nevius, L.W. from the Wellcome Collection. This work is in the public domain in the United States because it was published (or registered with the U.S. Copyright office) before January 1, 1925.

Fig. 6-3: (Wooden statue of stomach operation, Cameroon, 1925): From the Science Museum, London and the Wellcome Collection, Attribution 4.0 International (CC BY 4.0).

Fig. 6-4: (percussion revolver): H. Holland, from Wikimedia Commons. In the public domain under Creative Commons Attribution 4.0 International License.

Fig. 6-5: (High-throughput screening device): Tiia Monto, from Wikimedia Commons. In the public domain though the Creative Commons Attribution-Share Alike 3.0 Unported License.

SELECTED BIBLIOGRAPHY

Barash, P.G. et al.: *Clinical Anesthesia Fundamentals.* Wolters Kluwer Health, first edition, 2015.

Funayama, S. and Cordell, G.A.: *Alkaloids.* Academic Press, 1 edition, 2014.

Hall, B.A. and Chantigian, R.C.: *Anesthesia: A Comprehensive Review.* Elsevier, 6th edition, 2019.

Martin, T.R.: *Ancient Greece.* Yale University Press, 2nd edition, 2013.

Mendelson, W.B.: *The Science of Sleep,* The University of Chicago Press, Chicago, 2017.

Mendelson, W.B.: *Understanding Sleeping Pills.* Independently published, 2018.

Mendelson, W.B.: *The Curious History of Medicines in Psychiatry,* Pythagoras Press, New York, 2020.

Mendelson, W.B.: *Molecules, Madness, and Malaria: How Victorian Fabric Dyes Evolved into Modern Medicines for Mental Illness and Infectious Disease.* Pythagoras Press, New York, 2020.

Vinten-Johansen, P. et al.: *Cholera, Chloroform and the Science of Medicine: A Life of John Snow.* Oxford University Press, 1 edition, 2003.

REFERENCES

[1] William Morton's life is described in a number of sources. Among them are: Martin, R.F., Wasan A.D., and Desai, S.: An appraisal of William Thomas Green Morton's life as a narcissistic personality. Anesthesiology 117: 10-14, 2012. Accessed online July 18, 2020. doi: https://doi.org/10.1097/ALN.0b013e31825922e1   Also see: Adams, A.K.: Review of 'Tarnished idol: William Thomas Green Morton and the Introduction of surgical anesthesia. *Journal of the Royal Society of Medicine* 95: 266-267, 2002. Accessed online July 18, 2020. https://www.ncbi.nlm.nih.gov/pmc/articles/PMC1279690/

[2] Fitzharris, L.: How ether transformed surgery from a race against the clock. *Scientific American* online, October 1, 2017. Accessed July 20, 2020. https://www.scientificamerican.com/article/how-ether-transformed-surgery-from-a-race-against-the-clock/

[3] Mendelson, W.B.: *The Science of Sleep.* University of Chicago Press, Chicago, 2017.

[4] See Mendelson, W.B. 2017, above.

[5] Brown, E.N., Lydic, R. and Schiff, N.D.: General anesthesia, sleep, and coma. *New England Journal of Medicine,* 363(27): 2638–2650, 2010. doi:10.1056/NEJMra0808281

[6] Hagihira, S.: Changes in the electroencephalogram during anaesthesia and their physiological basis. *Brit. J. Anesthesia* 115, suppl. 1: i27-i31, 2015. https://doi.org/10.1093/bja/aev212

[7] Vacas, S.: Sleep and anesthesia—common mechanisms of action. Sleep Med. Clin. 8: 1-9, 2013. Accessed July 17, 2020. doi: 10.1016/j.jsmc.2012.11.009

[8] Mendelson, W.B.: *Molecules, Madness, and Malaria: How Victorian fabric dyes evolved into modern medicines for mental illness and infectious disease.* Pythagoras Press, New York, 2020a.

[9] Escohotado, A.: A Brief History of Drugs: From the Stone Age to the Stoned Age. Park Street Press, Rochester, Vermont, 1999.

[10] See Escohotado, A., 1999 above.

[11] See Escohotado, A., 1999 above.

[12] See Escohotado, A., 1999 above.

[13] Etymology online dictionary (Etymonline.com): pharmacy, accessed 7/8/20.

https://www.etymonline.com/word/pharmacy

[14] Smith, W.D. in *Encyclopedia Britannica* online. Accessed July 24, 2020.

https://www.britannica.com/biography/Hippocrates

[15] Astyrakaki, E. et al.: References to anesthesia, pain, and analgesia in the Hippocratic Collection. Anesth. Analg. 110: 188-194, 2010. doi: 10.1213/ane.0b013e3181b188c2

[16] Hargrave, J.C. in *Encyclopedia Britannica* online: Paracelsus. Accessed July 24, 2020.

https://www.britannica.com/biography/Paracelsus

[17] Alexander, J.C. and Joshi, G.P.: A review of the anesthetic implications of marijuana use. Proc (Bayl Univ Med Cent) 32: 364-371, 2019. Accessed July 27, 2020. doi: 10.1080/08998280.2019.1603034

[18] James, S.: *A Clinician's Guide to Cannabinoid Science.* Cambridge University Press, Cambridge UK, in press.

[19] Nicholson, A.N. et al.: Effect of D-9-Tetrahydrocannabinol and Cannabidiol on Nocturnal Sleep and Early-Morning Behavior in

Young Adults. *J Clin Psychopharmacol* 24:305–313, 2004. https://mail.google.com/mail/u/0/#inbox/WhctKJVRKDzKZJVXtBgJlbtC kplXlVhjnbqBZbwfBcRfgnCbMFwsKPFKfCQvMJJVhHXcpJq?projector=1 &messagePartId=0.1.1

[20] Babson, K.A. et al.: Cannabis, Cannabinoids, and Sleep: A Review of the Literature. Curr Psychiatry Rep 19, 23 (2017). https://doi.org/10.1007/s11920-017-0775-9

[21] National Academies of sciences, engineering and medicine: The health effects of cannabis and cannabinoids. The National Academies Press, Washington, D.C., 2017. doi: https://doi.org/10.17226/24625

[22] Babson, K.A., Sottile, J. and Morabito, D.: Cannabis, cannabinoids, and sleep: a review of the literature. Current Psychiatry Reports 19, 2017 online. Accessed August 1, 2020. https://link.springer.com/article/10.1007/s11920-017-0775-9

[23] Sznitman, S.R. et al.: Medical cannabis and insomnia in older adults with chronic pain: a cross-sectional study. *BMJ Supportive & Palliative Care.* Published Online First: 20 January 2020. doi: 10.1136/bmjspcare-2019-001938

[24] Whitby, J.D.: Alcohol in anesthesia and surgical resuscitation. *Anesthesia* 35: 502-505, 1980. https://onlinelibrary.wiley.com/doi/pdf/10.1111/j.1365-2044.1980.tb03830.x

[25] Landholdt, H-P and Gillin, J.C.: Sleep abnormalities during abstinence in alcohol-dependent patients. *CNS Drugs* 15: 413-425, 2001. https://doi.org/10.2165/00023210-200115050-00006

[26] Karp, M. and Sokol, J.K.: Intravenous use of alcohol in the surgical patient. *JAMA* 146: 21-23, 1951. doi:10.1001/jama.1951.03670010025006

[27] Homer: The Odyssey, Book 4, translation by Ian Johnston, accessed July 9, 2020. http://www.hellenicaworld.com/Greece/Literature/Homer/en/Odyssey04.html

[28] Miller, M.B. et al.: Pain Intensity as a Moderator of the Association between Opioid Use and Insomnia Symptoms among Adults with Chronic Pain. Sleep Medicine 52: 98-102, 2018 https://doi.org/10.1016/j.sleep.2018.08.015

[29] Kay, D.C., Eisenstein, R.B., and Jasinski, D.R.: Morphine effects on human REM state, waking state and NREM sleep.

Psychopharmacologia 14: 404-416, 1969. Accessed July 25, 2020. https://doi.org/10.1007/BF00403581

[30] Kay, D.C. et al.: Opioid Effects on Computer-Derived Sleep and EEG Parameters in Nondependent Human Addicts. *Sleep* 2: 175-191, 1979. https://doi.org/10.1093/sleep/2.2.175

[31] Rosen, I.L. et al.: Chronic opioid therapy and sleep: an American Academy of Sleep Medicine position statement. *J. Clin. Sleep Med.* 15: 1671-1673, 2019. https://jcsm.aasm.org/doi/10.5664/jcsm.8062

[32] Klein, C.:10 things you may not know about Samuel Colt. History.com, Sept. 4, 2018, accessed July 27, 2020. https://www.history.com/news/10-things-you-may-not-know-about-samuel-colt

[33] See Astyrakaki, E et al. 2010, ref. 15 above.

[34] Advisory Board Daily Briefing, November 20, 2012: "The 'most important' NEJM article ever published." https://www.advisory.com/Daily-Briefing/2012/11/20/The-most-important-NEJM-article-ever-published Accessed June 26, 2020.

[35] Rachlin, W.: The forgotten man, Samuel Guthrie. *Am. J. Surgery* XXXIX, No. 1, online, accessed July 31, 2020.

https://www.americanjournalofsurgery.com/article/S0002-9610(38)90750-0/pdf

[36] Winters, R.W.: Accidental Medical Discoveries: How Tenacity and Pure Dumb Luck Changed the World. Skyhorse Publishing, New York, 2016. https://www.barnesandnoble.com/readouts/accidental-medical-discoveries-how-tenacity-and-pure-dumb-luck-changed-the-world/

[37] American Medical Biographies: Guthrie, Samuel, 1920. Online, accessed July 31, 2020
https://en.wikisource.org/wiki/American_Medical_Biographies/Guthrie,_Samuel

[38] Guthrie, D.: Centenary of chloroform anesthesia. *Brit. Med. J.* Nov. 1, 1947, p. 701. Accessed July 29, 2020.
https://www.bmj.com/content/2/4530/701

[39] O'Leary, A.J.: Who was the person who discovered chloroform for anaesthesia: was it Simpson or Waldie? Presidential address to Liverpool Society of Anaesthetists. Accessed July 29, 2020.
https://www.bjanaesthesia.org.uk/article/S0007-0912(17)49062-3/pdf

[40] See Mendelson, W.B. 2020a, reference 8 above.

[41] Mendelson, W.B.: *The Curious History of Medicines in Psychiatry.* Pythagoras Press, New York, 2020b.

[42] See Mendelson, W.B., 2020a, reference 8 above.

[43] See Mendelson, W.B., 2020b, reference 41 above.

[44] Dehn, L.: *The Real Tsaritsa.* Little Brown, Boston, 1922, p. 138.

[45] Susann, J.: *Valley of the Dolls: 50th anniversary edition.* Tiger LLC, sold on Amazon 2016.

[46] Memorial and Museum: Auschwitz-Birkenau online. Accessed July 30, 2020.
http://auschwitz.org/en/history/camp-hospitals/selections-and-lethal-injections/ See also Helm, S.: If this is a woman: Inside Ravensbruck. Abacus, London, 2015, pp. 243-358.

[47] Fuchs, H.: For third time this week, the federal government carries out an execution. *The New York Times* online, July 17,2002. Accessed July 18, 2002. https://www.nytimes.com/2020/07/17/us/dustin-honken-federal-execution.html?referringSource=articleShare

[48] Reuters: Special report: how the Trump administration secured a secret supply of execution drugs. *The New York Times* online July 10, 2020. Accessed July 18, 2020.

https://www.nytimes.com/2020/07/17/us/dustin-honken-federal-execution.html?referringSource=articleShare

[49] Iqbal, N. et al.: Ethylene role in plant growth, development and senescence: interaction with other phytohormones. *Front. Plant Sci.* April 4, 2017. Accessed July 30, 2020. https://doi.org/10.3389/fpls.2017.00475

[50] Dabbagh, A. and Rajaei, S.: Halothane: is there still any place for using the gas as an anesthetic? *Hepat Mon.* 11: 511-512, 2011 https://www.ncbi.nlm.nih.gov/pmc/articles/PMC3212768/

[51] World Nuclear Association: How is uranium made into nuclear fuel? Accessed July 24, 2020. https://www.world-nuclear.org/nuclear-essentials/how-is-uranium-made-into-nuclear-fuel.aspx

[52] O'Brien, H.D.: The introduction of halothane into clinical practice: the Oxford experience. *Anesthesia and Intensive Care.* 34, Suppl. 1,27-32, 2006. https://journals.sagepub.com/doi/pdf/10.1177/0310057X0603401S03

[53] See O'Brien, H.D. 2006, reference 52 above.

[54] See Mendelson, W.B. 2020b, reference 41 above.

[55] See Mendelson, W.B. 2020b, reference 41 above.

[56] See Mendelson, W.B. 2020b, reference 41 above.

[57] Makin, S.: Behind the Buzz: how ketamine changes the depressed patient's brain. *Scientific American*, April 12, 2019, accessed July 1, 2020. https://www.scientificamerican.com/article/behind-the-buzz-how-ketamine-changes-the-depressed-patients-brain/

[58] Acevedo-Diaz, EE. et al.: Comprehensive assessment of side effects associated with a single dose of ketamine in treatment-resistant depression. https://doi.org/10.1016/j.jad.2019.11.028 (link is external), Nov. 10, 2019, *Journal of Affective Disorders.*

[59] Escobar, A.: Propofol addiction. Drugaddictiontreatment.com, accessed July 4, 2020.
https://www.drugaddictiontreatment.com/types-of-addiction/prescription-drug-addiction/propofol-addiction/

[60] See Mendelson, W.B., 2017, reference 3 above.

[61] Tung, A., Lynch, J.P., and Mendelson, W.B.: Prolonged sedation with propofol in the rat does not result in sleep deprivation. *Anesth. Analg.* 92: 1232-1236, 2001.

[62] Tung,A.; Bergmann,B.; Herrera,S.; Cao,D.; Mendelson, W.B.: Recovery from sleep deprivation occurs during propofol anesthesia. *Anesthesiology* 100: 1419-1426, 2004.

[63] Miller, A.L., Theodor, D., and Widrich, J.: (updated May 18, 2020). StatPearls (Internet). StatPearls Publishing, Treasure Island, Florida. https://www.ncbi.nlm.nih.gov/books/NBK554540/#_NBK554540_pub det

[64] Burns, W.: Ross C. Terrell, an anesthetic pioneer. *Anesthesia Analgesia* 113: 387-389, 2011. doi: 10.1213/ANE.0b013e3182222b8a

[65] See Miller, A.L. et al. 2020, reference 63 above.

[66] Mason KP et al.: Effects of dexmedetomidine sedation on the EEG in children. *Paediatric Anaesthesia.* 2009 Dec;19(12):1175–1183. DOI: 10.1111/j.1460-9592.2009.03160.x

[67] Wu, X-H et al.: Low-dose dexmedetomidine improves sleep quality pattern in elderly patients after noncardiac surgery in the intensive care unit: a pilot randomized controlled trial. *Anesthesiology* 125: 975-991, 2016. https://pubmed.ncbi.nlm.nih.gov/27571256/

[68] Miranda, G.A., Krystal, A.D. and Fierro, AM.A.: Nocturnal dexmedetomidine in non-intubated, critically ill patients: sleep or sedation? *Anesthesiology* 127: 397-398, 2017. https://pubmed.ncbi.nlm.nih.gov/28719531/
Also see Reel, B. and Maani, C.V.: Dexmedetomidine. StatPearls, February 21, 2020. Accessed July 4, 2020. https://www.ncbi.nlm.nih.gov/books/NBK513303/

[69] Holbrook, A.M. et al.: A meta-analysis of benzodiazepines in the treatment of insomnia. CMAJ 162: 225-233, 2000.
https://pubmed.ncbi.nlm.nih.gov/10674059/

[70] NICE: Guidance on the use of zaleplon, zolpidem and zopiclone for the short-term management of insomnia | Guidance | NICE. (NICE concluded no significant difference in Z drugs and benzodiazepines in terms of efficacy or safety). 2004.
https://www.nice.org.uk/guidance/ta77

[71] Niroshan Siriwardena, A. et al.: Magic bullets for insomnia? Patients' use and experiences of newer (Z drugs) versus older (benzodiazepine) hypnotics for sleep problems in primary care. Brit. J. General Practice 58: 417-422, 2008. DOI:
https://doi.org/10.3399/bjgp08X299290

[72] Agravat, A.: 'Z'-hypnotics versus benzodiazepines for the treatment of insomnia. *Prog. Neurol. Psychiat.* 22 Vol 22 Iss. 2 2018, pp. 26-29 online. Accessed July 19, 2020.
https://onlinelibrary.wiley.com/doi/epdf/10.1002/pnp.502

[73] Hoffmann, F.: Benefits and risks of benzodiazepines and Z drugs: comparison of perceptions of GPs and community pharmacists in Germany. Ger Med Sci v.11; 2013, accessed July 15, 2020.
https://www.ncbi.nlm.nih.gov/pmc/articles/PMC3728643/

[74] Air Force Special Operations Command Instruction 48-101, archived June 11, 2014 at the Wayback Machine, U.S. Air Force Special Operations command, November 30, 2012.

[75] Mendelson, W.B.: *Understanding Sleeping Pills.* Independent, 2018.
https://www.amazon.com/Understanding-Sleeping-Pills-Wallace-Mendelson/dp/1718039980/ref=sr_1_1?dchild=1&keywords=Understanding+sleeping+pills&qid=1594914490&sr=8-1

[76] See Mendelson, W.B. 2020a, reference 8 above.

[77] 2018 Lasker-DeBakey Clinical Medical Research Award: Discovery and development of propofol, a widely used anesthetic. Accessed July 14, 2020.
http://www.laskerfoundation.org/awards/show/discovery-and-development-propofol-widely-used-anesthetic/

[78] See Mendelson, W.B. 2020b, reference 41 above.

[79] See Mendelson, W.B. 2020b, reference 41 above.

[80] Wouters, O.J., McKee, M., and Luyten, J.: Estimated research and development investment needed to bring a new medicine to market, 2009-2018. JAMA 323: 844-853, 2020. doi:10.1001/jama.2020.1166

[81] See Mendelson, W.B. 2020b, reference 41 above.